Fit as a Fiddle
Happy as a Lark

Fit as a Fiddle
Happy as a Lark

A Guide to Physical & Mental Wellbeing

Neelam Mankar

Sreeti A Amonkar

Fit as a Fiddle Happy as a Lark

Table of Contents

About the Authors

Could there be an any better moment for this book to come out? I think not. We are rendered with an unprecedented situation.

The capricious virus bodes ill for those who aren't attuned to their wellbeing. And being so, our surest bet in the fight against this pandemic with unmitigated transmogrification is our robust health- both mental and physical. Hence, the subject was chosen for this book.

We all know that this too shall pass and, in its passing, the humanity shall be left with an irreversible alteration made to their daily lives which, if employed to our advantage may work wonder for us.

The book that you are holding in your hands shall prove to be instrumental in this quest for maintaining or regaining your well-being.

Neelam Mankar, the author of "Fit as a Fiddle" is a fitness enthusiast who has lived a life committed to health, wealth, and good relations. This commitment has taken her through some amazing memories, both, personally and professionally. Working for thirty-four years in a prestigious government organisation, viz. Reserve Bank of India and National Bank of Agriculture & Development, has made her an expert Financial Coach. Abundance is one of her foremost values and she believes in creating an abundant life for herself and her clients. She is also a Certified Life Coach.

A globe-trotter at heart, she has travelled to 24 countries. One of the motivations in all her visits has been to explore the fitness and wellness culture around the world. Keeping herself updated with new and upcoming fitness trends has been a relentless pursuit for her.

Neelam's achievements say it all. Though she is in her golden years, in 2019 she effortlessly conquered the Tiger's Nest in Bhutan, which even a person in their twenties would find difficult. In 2018, she took part in the Guinness Book of records Plankathon event held in Pune, India. One must say, a person who has lived as good as without a single pill all her life surely has earned the right to write a book on health. I have known Neelam for a couple of years now and I can assure you that she practises what she preaches.

Talking about Sreeti A. Amonkar, the author of "Happy as a Lark", with over twenty-five years of broad experience under her belt, she is hailed as one of the foremost communication skills trainers in the industry right now. One has to only Google her out to read about all the remarkable things that her students, clients and ex-employers have to say about her.

What allured her to visit Bhutan in 2019 was to meet the citizens of the world's happiest nation. Her happiness knew no bounds, the very moment she stepped onto the land of happiness. Her take on the entire visit to Bhutan was that material possessions hardly constitute for real happiness.

I have known Sreeti for quite a few years now. It's not that her life is perfect. On the contrary, just like everybody else's, she has her share of joys and sorrows. What sets her apart is that she always exudes happiness. Her happiness is contagious. That's why I feel she is the best person to write on the subject of happiness. I'm sure that this contagion of happiness will be passed on to you by the time you are done reading this book.

I'm in awe of the sheer thoughtfulness with which this book has been written and I consider it my privilege to write an introduction to these two wonderful women, who have never stopped inspiring me. I sincerely hope that you will find this book as useful as it has been for me.

-Prashant Krushna Prakash Sonawane
Pune, Maharashtra
Dakini Day
17th May, 2020

Foreword

Being an obesity specialist with a keen interest in child obesity, I've spent a considerable part of the last 10 years trying to connect the dots as to the origins of this insidious intruder.

I now regularly see obese, low self-esteemed 12-15-year olds with an expanded dictionary including A for anxiety, B for Bipolar, D for Depression and so on. Every mother walks in suggesting her obese 9 year old daughter has a thyroid problem or some metabolic disorder, it's never the food or exercise at fault.

Initially I used blackmail, the whole negative psychology approach such as "Don't worry about this child's future, as he/she won't live long enough to have one" …. or "you need to worry about yourself as you will most probably outlive your child".

Higher level work began. Slightly more subtle approaches; I watched parents become aghast when confronted with the suggestions that these children are simply mirroring their own personalities. They were a sum total of their parent's paradoxes and poor coping mechanisms. At some point I had to shift the blame.

Appears we as parents are in a hurry for our children to age, to sound more and more adult-ish sooner. We pride ourselves on their ability to read books, solve mathematical puzzles, converse using polysyllabic words on topics ranging from National Geographic, organic chemistry to online dramas, all in one breath. To quote a famous country music song "For everything you win there's something lost" So what's this generation losing?

My mind gets tempted by the clichés of innocence, health and the ability to make offline relationships. If only it were that simple. The answers had to be found, as being both a parent and a healer, the need to dig deeper bore weight, and I began the search.

 For starters they and by default we are accelerating towards mortality faster than any other generation in history. Life expectancy is at an all-time low if adjusted for drug supported living.

While grandparents born in the 40's and 50's remaining thin, became diabetic in their 70's , the next generation born in the 60's and 70's began experiencing these maladies in their 50's , it appears everyone born in the 80's and after are sitting in their 30's in waiting rooms asking questions linked to a new brand of "lifestyle diseases". Not to mention the allure of mental health that has captured the imagination of the youth around the globe.

When I dug deeper to look for possible causes and solutions it involved some introspection. I looked back at my youth, the ease with which we respected our elders, fought and patched up with our mates, ate homemade junk and yes, played a lot of sports. We spent hours finding our own values, finding joy and accumulated knowledge enroute. Using them as a map or an anchor to live out our lives. Somewhere along the way guided by these values retreating to them as a mariner would to a compass, we retained optimism, humour even, built resilient minds and bodies, even in the face of adversities. Finding happiness besides our professional and personal responsibilities.

The question each of us needs to answer is one of identity. For example, when I'm not with patients, I'm a triathlete either in the pool, on the bike or on a run. When I'm not parenting or being a dutiful husband or son, I'm reading or writing. I often play the guitar too. I've reached a conclusion, having non-commercial hobbies don't make me irresponsible or indulgent. Hobbies both physical and mental, anchor me when things go awry. It's taken quite a few knocks along the way to get to where I have. 18 fractures, 9 surgeries, most under general anaesthesia and yes, a chronic illness despite which, I choose to pursue betterment in my chosen roles.

So why then do we need to invest time in reading about lifestyle and wellness?

As we go through the years, I wonder are we consuming or are we being consumed? Are we the ones spending or getting spent? The word investment appears to have an almost transactional, financial undertone.

The issue at hand, often the unspeakable is one of graceful ageing. How do we bravely traverse the mine filled path that awaits us? This demands urgency barring which choices get taken for us and life becomes mostly reactive.

Must we spend our days reacting to existential emergencies? Or oscillating between extremes of despair and bliss?

Often it is inspiration we seek. I find the easiest call to action to stir us out of learned helplessness or inertia is a moment of connection. To a fertile mind a well worded metaphor often does the trick to bring on a few years of stimulated learning and living. Then onto the next. I find each decade may have it's own trigger. I hope this book helps fill a void. Connect with the authors, feel their intentions, go beyond the knowledge, open yourself up, and liberate the scepticism of having heard it all before. Just be.

It's time for some of us to step up and chronicle journeys and possible technical and emotional pathways to living out our potentials.

Sreeti and Neelam are evolved souls to have taken on the time and responsibility to redraw the map. More importantly help us redraw our own. Use the diet, exercise and stress management principles highlighted to remember your youthful days, before words like stress, diet, obesity and unfulfilled expectations became part of our vocabulary. Beyond a to – do model, it is more a DIY (Do It Yourself) …

Both authors through their life experiences have presented unique perspectives on their journeys. Let me not delay it further. Let your journey begin.

-Dr. Malhar Hamir Ganla
Pune, Maharashtra

Acknowledgements

We would like to acknowledge all the people who have helped directly or indirectly in writing this book. However, some contributors deserve a special mention.

A special thanks to our mentor, Mr Arfeen Khan, under whose guidance we have written this book in such a short period.

Dr Malhar Ganla, a dear friend of ours, is the first person who came to our mind when we thought of seeking a foreword for our book. Dr Ganla is a Consulting Clinical Exercise Psychologist and a Certified Triathlon Coach. To our great delight, he was more than happy to oblige.

It would have been impossible without the consistent guidance and insights from Mr Prashant Sonawane, who is no less than a family to both of us. He is a Corporate Trainer, and an Independent Researcher in Buddhist Philosophy. We especially loved the title he came up with for this book.

We are grateful to our beloved friend Mr Bhavin Patel for designing our book despite his extremely busy schedule. Mr Patel is an IT expert and an entrepreneur who is featured as a thought leader in several prestigious magazines.

Last but not the least, we would like to express our gratitude to Mr Kishor Chobhe, a businessman, author, coach and most of all a very good friend of ours. In spite of his hectic schedule, Mr Chobhe extended his support in the technical aspects of publishing.

We hope that this book satisfies the purpose for which you have picked it up. We wish you happy reading and most of all a healthy and happy life.

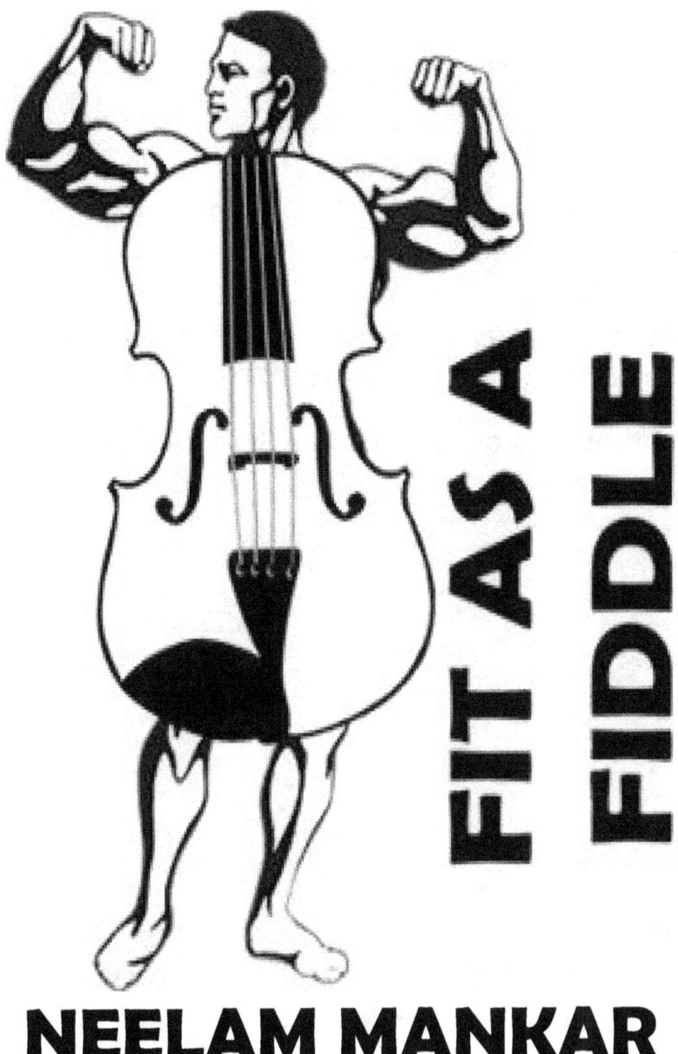
FIT AS A
FIDDLE
NEELAM MANKAR

Dedication

I would like to dedicate this book to my family, my sister Bijoly Latkar and my sons Sandesh & Rajeev, who have been so loving and caring and continue to be my world. A special dedication to Papa, my dear grandfather, without whom I would not be the person today I am.

Last but not the least our dear Golden Retriever, Sheron a darling of our family.

Introduction

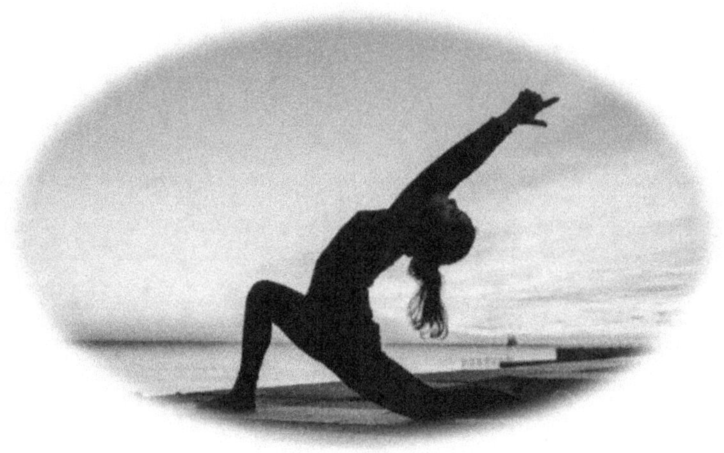

"Health is a state of complete mental, social and physical well-being, not merely the absence of disease or infirmity"

-World Health Organization, 1948

"Health is Wealth", the adage heard time and again, especially when one gets unwell, a reminder to take care of one's health before anything else. So true! who else than me can agree with it, a woman who lived by it day in and day out. I, therefore, would like to express my need to share my story, a story of a woman who has led a healthy and active life throughout and continue to live the same, a life of energy and enthusiasm even in her 60's.

I am a senior citizen in my 60's as I mentioned above, retired from an active service of 34 years in a premium government organisation, viz, "National Bank for Agriculture and Rural Development, an organisation dedicated to the socio-economic development of India.

Throughout my life I have lived a healthy, wealthy and most importantly an active life. I owe this to my dear grandfather "Papa" as we called him dearly, who laid the foundation of the person today I am. He consistently motivated and inspired me to lead a social life, most importantly to be always ahead and be a part of various activities, conducted in school as well as in social clubs. These platforms groomed me into a self-confident, expressive and fearless person who loved to try challenges throughout her life. This attitude resulted in learning multi-activities such as swimming, horse riding, calisthenics, dancing, baseball and many more. Public speaking has become my forte, as stage fear is unknown to me. My passion to try different activities resulted in venturing from one form of exercise to another activity, when the present one would become effortless as I needed a higher challenge to meet my intense desire to stay fit and always in form. This journey gave me an opportunity to learn different forms of exercise, from yoga to aerobics. Cycling and walking was a regular part of my life. I feel blessed to have been given this inner desire to stay active and healthy. Consistency and sincerity played a key role in this endeavour of mine.

My high energy level and enthusiasm always attracted me to various adventurous sports, especially in last three decades. I always wanted every year of mine to be special, so made it a point to visit places in India and other countries, wherein I would get opportunities to try something new, such as a difficult hike, or a water sport like scuba diving or just go through certain wild forest to get a view of animals, so on and so forth. My fascination for wild animals took me to a number of wild forests, giving me an opportunity to get to see animals such lions, tigers, panthers, etc. and even Orangutans in Sarawak forest of Malaysia. Today in my 60's, I continue to participate in adventurous sports. Lately in 2018, I participated in a Guinness Book of World Records event "Plankathon", an event held in Pune, Maharashtra, India to break the earlier record held by China. In this event about 3000 persons collectively participated to hold the position of a plank for 60 seconds simultaneously. I feel proud to have been a part of this great event, which has made India the present holder of this record. Further, last year, that is in 2019, I visited Bhutan and climbed the mountain "Tiger's Nest". Some of you may have climbed this mountain and seen how difficult the trek is, as the Bhutan government has kept its natural form, with its rocky formations and slippery slopes. This trek I completed after both of my knees were replaced. Sounds astounding right? No, I don't think anyone should, as you may have heard of several persons with disabilities climbing the Himalayas. From where did this confidence come from, simple! my belief in myself and the self-confidence. I do not intend to impress you with my list of achievements, its only to express the power of such achievements in one's life. It gives you that extra dose of energy, happiness and above all the feeling of good factor in one's life. Isn't it so satisfying that I have lived every moment with so much of zest and energy and have no regret? Time is the most important commodity of our life and years pass by without us knowing so quickly. Avail of the opportunities thrown to you and make life a journey of wonderful life achieving moments, you can reflect on in your sunset years. It will make one happy of leading a fulfilling life.

 Our childhood has a profound effect on our thinking and the lifestyle we desire. However, as we grow older and gain experience our perspective to life changes. The lifestyle we lead has a snowball effect, over the years positive or negative. The same thing happened to me. Consistency and persistence to my commitment to good health had a snowball effect in my 50's. It was like my new birth and new interests. An age when people start slowing down, I was venturing into various awe-inspiring sports like night hikes, braving through rough seas to visit the Amazon Rainforest in Brazil and Sarawak forest in Borneo, Malaysia, and many more. It is said life begins at 50 and sure it does. I am a living example. My real life began at 50 and it continuous to be an amazing, beautiful journey. And my sincere wishes for all my readers to lead a life, which you can proudly look back on.

Health: A Perspective

"I believe that the greatest gift you can give your family and the world is a healthy you."
                                        -Joyce Mayer

Whenever you meet someone after a long time or speak to someone after a gap of several days, several months or several years, the conversation starts with a question "How are you? How is your health? These questions randomly used truly indicate, that on everyone's mind health is predominant. Health is the first concern of each one of us. Health forms an important pillar of our lives. We may have all the luxuries in life, however, to enjoy them good health is a pre-requisite. Good health, obviously plays a key role in our holistic happiness. Yet, how many of us give its importance it deserves? Negligible few.

We are presently living in a world of extravaganza. Variety has become the spice of life and indulgence in rich, lip-smacking dishes has become a norm of the day. Today, we are living in a fast-paced world with rapid changes in the material world, from electronics to fast foods. Most of us are rushing to earn the maximum we can, leaving either no time or less time to cook our own meals or exercise our bodies. We are leading a sedentary life, abusing our bodies by stuffing in fast food to satisfy our hunger and taste and most importantly not giving the body the opportunity to burn those extra calories. The world is facing several deadly diseases due to these modern unhealthy lifestyles, such as heart problems, diabetes, cancer, blood pressure, etc. And the irony is that, the wake-up call arises when the disease has been detected at a fairly high stage.

To withstand the storms of life-threatening diseases, there is a dire need for change in our lifestyle, in our diet and obviously added to that, introduction of some regular exercise in our day-to-day life routine, as the saying goes "Prevention is better than cure". However, it's heartening to know that, some of you may be leading a healthy life, with some form of exercise routine and staying focused to your health. Hearty congratulations to you all. However, there may be some of you who are leading a sedentary life not by choice though, but by compulsion. Some of you may be fit and fine having an edge of youth despite leading a sedentary life. Lucky you, however, we all know that luck is occasional and can never be relied on. Reflection on one's health status and it's need to satisfy our body needs and thus workout some workable program to stay away from ill-health in future is not ruled out. You may be feeling why I am reiterating the same thing repeatedly and urging you so strongly to redesign your daily schedule to incorporate a meticulous exercise plan? A very simple reason, we all are blessed with such a beautiful body to enjoy the fruits of this universe and its our moral duty to keep it healthy and fit and most importantly in our self-interest.

 Life is a blessing, I valued it and I continue to value it. Despite being in my 60's I wish to continue living on the same plane and by God's grace may live for another 2 to 3 decades. I want to see the world and enjoy the beautiful moments it has to offer. My vision to see this world as a beautiful place of healthy and wealthy people can be attained through my mission as a Life coach and a Finance coach.

When one talks of health, it may convey a number of perspectives. Each one of us attaches a different meaning to it. For some. it may mean "I am fit and fine as I am able to perform at my work", for some it may mean "I have a good enviable figure", for some "Being healthy may mean being plump and not skinny", so on and so forth. So, what does healthy mean? Healthy in a lay man's language can be said as a state, wherein it allows a person to cope with all demands of daily life. It can also be said as a physical, mental and social wellbeing and as a resource for living a full life. It refers not only to the absence of disease, but the ability to recover and bounce back from illness and other problems.

"The doctor of the future will give no medicine, but will interest his patients in the care of the human frame, in diet and in the cause and prevention of disease."
                                        - Thomas Edison

Being healthy gives freedom in almost every area of life. My experience endorses this statement. I lived all my life as good as, without a pill. For this I am extremely grateful to the Universe, for guiding me in a right direction towards health and wealth. Though partially, I can give credit to myself, for staying committed and inspired all my life. In this regard, I am extremely grateful for my values, that luckily aligned with the activities I loved to do. Activities when aligned with our highest values, do not need any inspiration to do them. The person just loves doing it. Values are developed from our childhood, through parents, grandparents, relatives, teachers, friends and whomever you come in close contact with. To quote a few of the values developed since childhood, they are family, love, integrity, happiness, appreciation, acclamation, abundance, peace, perfection, so on and so forth. The list can go very long. However, we all have certain values developed and some of them will be highest on our priority list. When a person does something congruent to his highest values, he or she enjoys it, as a result performs well. We all have a list of values, and if any action is performed in alignment with our highest values, the action is carried out with joy and effortlessly. In my case, my eating habits and exercise choices were congruent with my highest values.

My highest values are abundance, love, family, appreciation and admiration. I lived an abundant life, loving and appreciating my body, always considered it as a God given gift. My well-maintained figure was admired and appreciated. This kept me inspired. I don't like monotony, so I kept on making changes in my form of exercise and over and above it, it helped me to take my exercises to a higher level. Values can be discovered through a value determination process. During my Life coaching and Finance coaching, I help my clients to discover their values, as it forms the foundation for success in any field of your life, be it physical, financial, emotional, mental or spiritual. And most importantly, they can be used as a guiding tool to take decisions on any aspect of our life. To give a kick start the journey towards a healthy body, a basic 4-step strategy is suggested, which can assist in achieving the desired outcome.

Chapter One

The Journey Begins

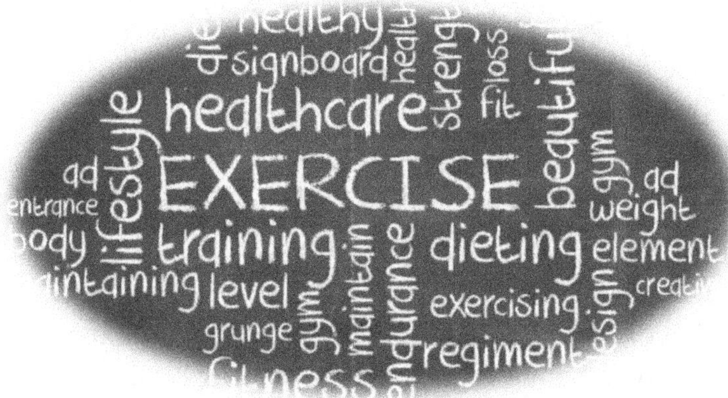

"You don't have to be great to start, but you have to start to be great"

-Zig Ziglar

"The secret of getting ahead is getting started"

-Mark Twain

Step 1: Decision Making

To achieve any outcome, be it physical or financial, the first step is initiation from our side, a firm decision to go ahead to achieve the desired outcome with sincerity and commitment. The decision once taken, sets one on this wonderful transformational journey. As I mentioned before, we have developed certain values since childhood and for all we know, they may not be complementing our goal. In view of this, we need to unlearn and relearn certain tools that will help us move towards our goal and start the journey in earnestness. Further, the point to understand is that we may have cultivated certain dietary habits that have led you to become the person you are today. Some of these habits too may or may not compliment your journey ahead. Some of these habits may require slight changes or may even require drastic changes, in case you are fond of and regularly eat rich, heavy, high cholesterol food.

Today we come across a number of exotic diets, either to stay healthy and fit or reduce weight. Given a choice, I always preferred a normal home food as it gave me the comfort of good, healthy food. Flexibility is the key to enjoyment, so I also enjoyed a variety of food outside occasionally. However, whenever you have your food from outside, eating in moderation always keeps you happy, satisfied and most importantly stay in shape.

A firm decision is, therefore, the first crucial step which sets the ball rolling. Procrastination is the enemy to any action, and so should be guarded from. Most of us are used to living in a comfort zone, and therefore fear any change in it and prefer to continue in that zone. This very often leads to procrastination. Decision, therefore, takes courage, a strong will to bring a change in ourselves for the better. Very often, we see several people bring about a change in their dietary habits and exercise habits to reduce or bring about a change in their looks for some special occasion or maybe even under the influence of somebody. However, in such cases the purpose for which the change has taken place is a fickle one and not one that is worthwhile. As a result, such people go back to their original selves. A strong purpose, therefore, plays a very important role in our decision to embark on the journey of good health. Discovering your purpose will assist in taking a decision, that you will adhere to, whatever it takes. Decision taken is almost like the half battle won.

Step-2: A meticulous workable plan

A decision without a plan is futile. It's like day dreaming and wishing for the something to happen, which is near to impossible. To make your dream come true an action needs to be initiated, an action that will result in a plan. However, as we all know to design a plan, we need to gain knowledge and an insight into the subject and necessarily the outcome desired. To enable you to initiate action and prepare a practical, workable plan, information on the major concepts viz. diet, exercise and mindset have been given in following chapters. The information given is of general nature, as I am not a doctor or dietician. As I have been reiterating that my intention to write this book along with my co-author, is to spread the importance of good health, emotional as well as physical in one's life.

A few suggestions are given below, which may be used as guidelines to chalk out a practical and workable plan for a healthy body with a healthy positive mind:

First and foremost, any plan should start with the end in mind. The end result can vary from person to person, such as weight loss, attainment of a presentable figure, attainment of a normal healthy body to perform the best in one's day-to-day activities, etc.

Second, a review of the present state of your health, your dietary and exercise habits, any illness, etc. In this context, a useful tip, maintain a diary of the details of your daily intake of food with the time, along with the exercise routine if any for initially a week. In a week's time you will be in a position to get a realistic picture of your daily habits, habits that has made you the way you are today.

Third, in view of the information collected above, a detailed plan can be designed keeping the end in mind, the outcome you desire. As the management mantra goes, we should have SMART goals to achieve them successfully. The designed plan should also be a SMART goal, viz. specific, measurable, achievable, realistic and time bound. Hope it makes sense! Or else it will stay just as a plan, as you will not be in a position to take a regular concrete review, leading to confusion. Confusion breeds

failure, whereas clarity breeds success. A realistic plan will help you stay on track and as the progress is seen, you will stay motivated and inspired. Further, most of us know consistency is the key to success, so stay consistent and sincere.

 # Fourth step, to make it more convenient to get the desired outcome, it always works when you break down your main plan into bit size plans with specific deadlines. Each of this bit-size plan will take you closer to the end result, and most importantly keep you happy and contented with these small achievements. The task of reaching your end result will get easy and effortless, and keep you on the right track.

Fifth, Initiate Action and follow the plan religiously.

Sixth, Follow-up of the plan

- Maintain a daily diary.
- Monitor the progress weekly or fortnightly.
- Make changes if required. Be flexible.
- Do not be stringent with your plan. As you progress your body will give you good signals. You surely will feel good and energetic, if the plan suits you. No plan is right or wrong. All of us are unique in our own ways, our needs are unique, so just design a plan with you and only you in mind.

Step 3: Diet

Diet plays a very important role in our health condition. Our body needs all nutrients in proper proportions to function smoothly, without any road blocks. Therefore, when these nutrients are supplied to our body in either less quantities or more quantities, than its need, imbalance takes place and illness occurs. The earlier generations never went for any special diets or counted the intake of calories. Yet, they were healthy and truly strong. My grandma, my parents never went to a doctor all their life, all they had was good home balanced meal. The normal daily meal consisted of rice, roti's, vegetables, pickle, salad, dal and papad. All the dishes were cooked in moderate vegetable oil (No fuss about which oil is good and which is bad). Today, we have a variety of oils in the market, confusing us. Homemade ghee was taken quite generously, without any fear of putting on weight. Occasional fish or chicken or meat was cooked. Breakfast too was homemade. Milk and fruits were a must daily. The best part was nothing was bought readymade from outside. I still remember, I would come to spend my summer vacation at my grandma's home in the outskirts of Pune, now a suburb, a sought-after urban area. The beautiful house was a spacious bungalow in almost acre of land, today a dream for most of us. It had a mini orchard with mango, guava, papaya, sapodilla (chickoo) plantations and the area was beautified with multi coloured flower plants. Above all there were some leafy edible plants, which gave us the much-needed iron a nutrient necessary for blood circulation. There was a river close by, where me and my friend would go to have a nice picnic at its shore. The reason behind sharing this story is that for making my picnic enjoyable my dear grandma would give me pakodas (a fried snack – fritter) made of leaves of the Ajwain (also known as ajowan caraway, bishop's weed or carom), a plant having medicinal value, viz. it is good for curing cold and hence a blessing during cold weather. I just loved them and still enjoy it, as I too have this particular plant on my home terrace. I have picked up such great, healthy and tasty dishes from her and my mother-in-law, who too fortunately for me was a wonderful cook. All of us have had and learned such great recipes from our dear ones. Inclusion of such wonderful healthy recipes in our regular food will surely make our meal not just colourful and appealing to your taste, but also give a positive boost to our health. Ultimately, innovation plays a key role in adding spice to our life. Today, when I look back, I feel lucky to have been born in a country, viz. India, so rich and versatile known world over for its colourful culture and most importantly for its cuisine.

To elicit the best performance and to preserve energy and health, it is important to provide proper maintenance in the form of a well-balanced diet, regular exercise, adequate sleep and periods of relaxation. Only a combination of all these four essentials can result in good health and natural good looks. Taking these four pillars in mind, the following chapters are dedicated to them.

Well Balanced Diet

"Every day is another chance to get stronger, to eat better, to live healthier, and to be the best version of you"

-Anonymous

The body uses food energy for two main purposes. First, to power all the body functions that are essential for life and health, such as breathing, blood circulation, digestion and excretion. Secondly, to provide energy for all the work done by the body, that is any sort of physical activity, from maintaining body posture to taking part in any activity. If you have enrolled for a health club membership, you may have noticed the first thing that the trainer does is to take your Body Mass Index (BMI). BMI is most basic measure of obesity and is internationally accepted standard of measuring how overweight you are. It is calculated using your weight (in kilograms) and height (in square metres), and is independent of gender or age. It helps in identifying who is at risk of developing associated complications, such as heart disease, osteoarthritis, etc. BMI can be calculated by using the following formula:

BMI=Weight (kg) divided by Height (square of metres)

A table showing the relation between BMI and associated disease risk

Status	BMI	Disease Risk
Underweight	<18.5	
Normal	18.5 – 22.9	Increasing but acceptable risk
Overweight	23.0 – 24.9	Increased risk
Obesity I	25.0 – 29.9	High risk
Obesity II	>30.0	Higher risk

The above information can give you a fair idea, where you stand. It can assist you in designing an appropriate individual plan.

Further, here is some information on the normal quantity of calories required at various stages of life. Calories are a measure of the amount of energy contained in food. You use most of the calories you consume just to stay alive, to maintain your organs, and keep your muscles working. What makes one fat is not the calories, but consuming more calories in food than you need. The number of calories you use depends on your size, how long you exercise and the intensity of the activity. From about the age of 30, the metabolism slows down. Hence it is wise to reduce the calories slowly over the years there on.

Calories required per day at different stages of life:

- Growing Children – 1800 to 2200 calories
- Inactive Adults – Men – About 2400 calories
  Women – About 2000 calories
- Active Adults – Men About 2850 calories
  Women – About 2150 calories
- Later in Life - Men About 2200 calories
  Women – 1850 calories

Eating is one of life's pleasures, and the key to good living is to choose food that is both healthy and delicious, at the same time a well-balanced diet. A well-balanced diet nourishes the body with its basic needs and gives us the required energy to carry out our day-to-day activities with zest and enthusiasm. It's quite conflicting to make our food more pleasurable and well-balanced at the same time. Hence to have knowledge on the nutrients required by our body, will go a long way to stay on a balanced diet and live a life of good health and vitality. I not being a dietician, have given general information on the various nutrients required for good health and the requirement of calories in general for various types of individuals, depending on their gender, work, height and weight. As I have benefitted from good health throughout my life, I felt the need to spread the importance of good health in one's life. By the way, I never ever measured my food or controlled my hunger to stay fit and fine. All I did was eat in moderation and saw to it that I consume all the necessary foods required for my body. Fortunately for me, born in a family headed by highly educated grandfather, the food cooked was perfect for good health. Daily consumption of milk and fruit, especially banana was mandatory. And to add icing to the cake, post marriage too, the family I got married into was very particular about good food. Over the years of experience, I have come to know what food serves me best and hence always was able to take the appropriate decisions related to it.

Most of us are aware of what is good for our health and most importantly what suits best for us. In today's informative age, we come across various articles on food, keeping us updated on the subject. The secret, however, lies in being selective for using it for personal use. Since my young age, I have had this habit of observing anything that appeared good in others and emulating the same, though may appear weird to some. This wonderful habit helped me introduce some of the awe-inspiring things into my life that added value to my overall well-being. In our life we meet innumerable people, near and far. Most of them have something to offer us, something that can add value to some or the other aspect of our life. It can be anything from physical, emotional, mental or even financial. All it needs is some awareness and our keen interest of commitment towards self-development. Such an attitude itself brings you in contact with positive, self-growing people. It's the Law of Attraction that's work here, that is like attracts like.

"The best six doctors anywhere and no one can deny it are sunshine, water, rest, air, exercise and diet"
-Wayne Fields

A healthy person who is neither gaining or losing weight, is an indication that same amount of energy is used as the food consumed. We may not consume the same amount of food on a daily basis, however, that should not be of much concern as it is balanced on a long term. Today we have access to all the information on products that add to our body fat. Therefore, its easy to keep some control on their intake.

A well-balanced diet provides the correct amount of all the essential nutrients, major of which are proteins, carbohydrates, fats, fibre, minerals and vitamins. The components of food that are essential for health are like a jigsaw puzzle, one missing link and the effectiveness of the whole system is destroyed. The body's major need is energy and we can meet this need by consuming a mixture of proteins, fats and carbohydrates. There a strong interdependence of the nutrients our body needs, hence our diet should be balanced to the best of our knowledge. Ability to adapt to variations in the quality and quantity of the diet goes a long way to maintain good health. Eating variety of foods will ensure any nutrient deficiency of a particular food being compensated by another food. No single food can provide completely adequate nutrition. A balanced diet is the best insurance against deficiency of any nutrients, helping us to live a healthy and energetic life. Just to give you an idea of the purpose of each of them, I have shared some information on the vital nutrients required for our body's smooth functioning.

Proteins

Proteins are required for the manufacture and repair of tissues. Our tissues wear and tear daily, proteins helps in renewing the worn-out tissues. They also repair the injured and diseased tissues. This demand can be met by products like chicken, peanuts, eggs, milk, cheese, peas, etc.

Carbohydrates

Carbohydrates are the sugars, starches and fibres found in fruits, grains, vegetables and milk products. Carbohydrates main function is to provide energy. Nowadays, many people go for low carbohydrate diet as they wish to reduce their weight. Reducing the amount of carbohydrate, you eat is really just another way to cutting down calorie intake.

Fats

The main function of fats in the diet is as a source of energy. It provides palatability, a necessity to enjoy and relish our food. The amount though will depend from person to person and largely on the national and personal eating habits. Intake of fat if taken in excessive amounts will make one over-weight and therefore susceptible to heart attacks.

Fibre

We often come across various several media, mentioning the importance of fibre in our diet. Fibre cannot be digested; hence they are known as roughage or dietary fibre. They, however hold water in the waste products in the bowels, which makes stool soft and bulky and speeds the passage of the food through the digestive system. Intake of fibre along with adequate daily exercise and drinking plenty of water can prevent constipation and digestive disorders. Fresh vegetables provide not only a bounty of vitamins and minerals, but also are a good source of dietary fibre.

Calcium

Calcium makes our bones and teeth hard and strong. Its need, therefore is highest in childhood. However, its requirement continues throughout our life. Milk and milk products such as cheese and yogurt are excellent sources of calcium, the nutrient essential for strong bones. It is also available in small quantities in many other foods, such as fish, pulses, nuts, etc. Potatoes and sweet-corn also provide a lot of calcium. A diet rich in calcium along with weight-bearing exercise can prevent loss of bone tissue, this is particularly important to prevent Osteoporosis, especially for women after menopause. Cigarette smoking is linked with lower bone density and greater loss of bone mass with age, so it is advisable to either cut it down, or better still stop smoking completely. Anyways, we all are aware that cigarette smoking is harmful for our health.

Iron

Iron forms a part of the red pigment of blood, called haemoglobin. Haemoglobin carries oxygen from the lungs to the tissues and carbon dioxide to the waste products, in the opposite direction. Lack of iron in the red pigment of the blood results in Anaemia. The lower haemoglobin levels in the person results in lack of vitality. Leafy green vegetables and cabbage are rich in iron.

Other minerals play a key role in our overall health. Salt is a necessary ingredient of our food to bring taste to it. However, excess salt is linked with blood pressure. The chemical name for salt is sodium chloride, and it is sodium which is harmful when taken in excess. It is in our best interest to favour caution and restrict the amount of salt we use. My experience in this connection, proves it right. I was expecting my third son. The delivery date was just a week away. My baby boy had grown to full 8+ pounds, waiting to come out in this world. My blood pressure as a result had shot up quite high and I was not in a position to take medication to bring it to normal. The doctor, therefore, advised me to consume less salt till I delivered my baby. I did religiously follow his advice. My blood pressure came back to normal and I gave natural birth to a healthy 8.5 lbs baby boy, on the expected date. Salt, thus you see can have a great impact on our blood pressure. Some of us do indulge heavily in salty snacks, snacks are naturally salty to give that tangy taste. However, if had in moderation, we may be able to enjoy them as well as keeping our blood pressure in check.

Fluoride

Fluoride is found in water and tea. It is needed for the hard enamel on teeth, reducing the likelihood of dental decay, most importantly for children. For healthy teeth and gums, brushing teeth twice a day with a tooth paste containing fluoride can prevent decay of teeth.

Vitamins and Minerals

Vitamins and Minerals are important nutrients essential for good health, since they help the body to use the energy stored in food.

Vitamins are substances that your body needs to grow and develop normally. There are 13 vitamins your body needs. They are vitamins A, C, D, E, K, and the B vitamins (8 of them).

Vitamins are divided into two categories: Water soluble and Fat soluble.

The four fat-soluble vitamins, viz. Vitamin A, D, E & K are absorbed into body fat and stored in the liver and fatty tissue, for later use. Hence, they need not be consumed each day. If taken in excess, however, some fat-soluble vitamins can accumulate in toxic amounts.

Vitamin C and the eight Vitamin B are all water-soluble, meaning they dissolve in body fluid, and most of the excess is eliminated through sweat or urine. Hence, there is little concern about toxic overdose, however, they need to be replenished regularly. The only way to get them is through a daily balanced diet.

Minerals play a part in the maintenance of immune cells, in blood coagulation, in the synthesis of oxygen in the blood, in bone formation and numerous other functions. Some, such as calcium, phosphorous and magnesium are necessary in fairly large amounts. The need for others, known as trace minerals, is much smaller. The essential trace minerals include iron, zinc, fluoride and copper.

With a few exceptions (notably vitamin D and K), the human body cannot make its own vitamins or minerals, so they must be obtained from foods. A balanced diet will supply all the vitamins and minerals that are necessary to maintain good health. Fruits and vegetables are highly rich in vitamins, especially A, C and E, in minerals such as calcium, magnesium, potassium and in antioxidants, which offer protection against certain cancers and heart disease. Many also contain valuable phytochemicals, which protect against disease and give colour and flavour to foods. Meat, poultry and fish are rich in minerals, such as iron, zinc and magnesium and important B vitamin. The proteins in meat, fish, dairy products and eggs supply eight amino acids, which the body cannot synthesise itself. Oily fish contains omega-3 fatty acids, which protect against heart disease and strokes and help those with arthritis.

Vitamin D, the sunshine vitamin

The so-called sunshine vitamin, vitamin D is manufactured in the skin when it is exposed to the ultra-violet rays of the sun. Vitamin D has a pivotal role in the absorption and utilisation of calcium. Although, you can obtain it from food, most of the vitamin the body needs come from sunshine. The action of sunshine on the skin converts a chemical naturally present in the body into active vitamin D, which is why vitamin D is known as "the sunshine vitamin". Hence, it is important to get out and get some sunshine. It can work its magic to our skin, making vitamin D for our body.

The richest food sources of vitamin D are oily fish such as mackerel and sardines. It is also found in butter, margarine, most low-fat spreads, full-cream, breakfast cereals and eggs.

Bio-chemical partnership – vitamins and minerals

Although all vitamins and minerals influence one another, some have special bio-chemical partnerships that affect how well they are absorbed by the body.

Vitamin C enhances the absorption of iron, for example topping a bowl of iron rich cereal with strawberries – is an excellent source of vitamin C.

Other nutrient partners include:

Vitamin D with Calcium

Vitamin E with Selenium

Vitamin B12 and Folic-acid

Calcium and Magnesium

Supplements

In the recent years, it is observed supplements are being taken to provide adequate amounts of essential vitamins and minerals. For people who skip regular meals and have to rely on fast foods, supplements may be a necessity. Certain people who are susceptible to deficiencies can benefit from supplements of vitamins and minerals. Among these are the elderly, people taking certain medications, people recovering from major illness, pregnant and nursing women.

You don't have to spend a fortune on food to eat healthily. Seasonal vegetables and fruits can give the required nutrients, along with cereals, cottage cheese, fish, chicken & meat and many more. The Universe has blessed us with nature abundant with innumerable edible vegetables and fruits and nuts to choose from.

Some tips to healthy eating are given below:

- Avoid too much highly refined, over-processed food.
- Grains such as rice and wheat, when milled to make polished rice and white flour, there is a significant loss of both nutrients and fibre. Hence, unpolished rice and wheat coarsely ground is recommended to get maximum nutrients and fibre.
- Recently, brown rice has become quite popular among the health-conscious people. Brown rice

retains its outer layer of bran and contains more vitamins, minerals and fibre than the white rice.

Step – 4: Water, Hydrate your body adequately with this miracle liquid

Water is the single most important nutrient for our bodies. It is involved in every function of our bodies. It is said that, you can stay without food for five to seven weeks without food, but the average adult can last more than five days without water.

- Our body is about 70 percent water
- Our muscles are about 75 percent water
- Our brain cells are 85 percent water
- Our blood is approximately 82 percent water
- Our bones are about approximately 25 percent water

The above information proves that water is the single most important nutrient for our body. Yet how many of us give it the due importance? How many of us consciously drink the required quantity of water daily?

Water makes up two-thirds of the body's weight. The amount of water you need depends on your size, how active you are and how hot the weather is. Generally, everyone needs to drink 6 to 8 glasses of water. Water is the best drink to rehydrate the body. Water is needed to hydrate our body and its parts, to enable them to function normally. It is necessary for digestion and absorption of food and helps the elimination of waste products by the kidney. The body loses water through perspiration, urination and exhalation. Replenishing it will maintain the balance and help you stay healthy and disease free. Most people rely on thirst to tell them when to drink water. By this time your body has actually dehydrated to slight extent. This is the reason you should drink water at regular intervals. Dehydration can cause illnesses such as headaches, dizziness, lethargy and dry skin. Less consumption of water can also lead to kidney stones. Today a number of aerated drinks are available to suit everyone's taste. Presently, the high standard of living has attracted majority of them towards the aerated drinks. Some energy drinks are also available that gives an option to quench your thirst. The result is, intake of pure clean water is minimum and other drinks maximum. This, however, does have an adverse effect on our body. Nothing like drinking a bottle of pure clean water. By the way, how many of us quench our thirst buying a bottle of some good clean water instead of a bottle of aerated drink, when we are travelling?

An interesting experience related to this. I was travelling from Paris, France to Zurich, Switzerland. At the Paris airport, I felt thirsty and needed water to quench my thirst. In most parts of Europe, the tap water is good for consumption. However, being an Indian I was not comfortable to drink tap water at the airport. I thought of buying water, so asked for the price of a mini water bottle. To my surprise the cost was much more than a premium wine bottle of the same volume. So, I purchased the wine bottle and drank a glass of it. To my surprise, it did not quench my thirst, on the contrary it increased it and had to consume some water to wet my throat. A lesson learned, never underestimate the power of water.

Water benefits us even beyond smooth body functioning. It gives us a smooth skin, more flexibility as the joints glide easily during movement, keeps us away from headaches, back pain, dry skin, heartburn, constipation and also memory loss. As brain cells are 85% water, if they stay hydrated, they will function well and keep at bay memory loss, which is observed in aging people. Water, according to me can be said to be an anti-aging liquid. We keep trying various anti-aging products, when we have within our means, this miracle liquid "water" to our ready disposal. The only caution to be exercised, here, is to drink clean water.

Last few decades due to commercialisation and mushrooming of industries, the ground water is being polluted with chemicals and pesticides. The water available to us needs purification for our use. I remember in 1992, when I shifted to my new flat in the outskirts of Pune, the water we had access to was the ground water from the well dug in the compound. The water then was so pure, it did not require even ordinary filtration. The only thing I did was I stored the water in a copper container, before using it for consumption. Trust me it was just perfect for my family's health. In the earlier days people used indigenous ways to purify water and stayed healthy and disease-free. One of the methods adopted during those days was, people stored water in copper containers. Today we have started using this method. We find in the market copper glasses, copper bottles and most importantly it has become popular even in the international market, because of its benefits. In India I have observed in many health- conscious households, water is stored in copper containers for consumption. It is said, that drinking water from copper containers helps our immune system, aids digestion, and has many more advantages.

Further, drinking appropriate quantity of quality water, goes a long way in maintaining a superb health. Some useful tips are given below:

- ✓ Start your day with a glass of water, preferably warm water
- ✓ Drink at least eight glasses of water daily
- ✓ Drink water about thirty minutes before meals or two hours after meals
- ✓ Drink room temperature water
- ✓ Do not drink much water after 7 pm, as it can interfere with your sleep
- ✓ Do not wait to feel thirsty to drink water, keep on drinking some water at regular intervals

Heart & Planning Meals for the Heart

"When the heart is at ease, the body is healthy"
                                            -Chinese proverb.

The heart is the strongest muscle in the body. It pumps tirelessly, moving the blood around the entire body via the network of arteries and capillaries and receiving blood back through the veins. Blood carries life-giving oxygen and nutrients around the muscular, elastic blood vessels to every cell in the body and takes away waste products such as carbon-dioxide. It is, therefore, absolutely necessary to protect them from any damage. Our diet will help us in this requirement. Time to take a fresh look into our overall eating habits. A moderate diet will keep it in good form.

 A type of fat, Cholesterol, has several functions in our body. There are two kinds of cholesterol, the cholesterol in the blood and cholesterol in food. However, let's not go into the technicalities. We basically need to know that excessive blood cholesterol poses a risk to your heart. You can use your diet to help prevent this from happening. There is good cholesterol and bad cholesterol. Good cholesterol helps to fight bad cholesterol. In view of this, intake of good cholesterol foods becomes a must to keep our heart happy and healthy. While foods that are high in cholesterol should be eaten in moderation, you needn't cut them out of your diet altogether, as the cholesterol they contain is broken down in our body relatively easily. One of the best things you can do for your heart is to shed any excess weight. Do this by eating a healthy, balanced, low-fat diet and by taking regular exercise. Physical activities, such as a brisk twenty minute walk each day has a dual benefit. Firstly, it helps to shed unwanted weight and secondly it protects us from heart disease by improving the efficiency of the heart and lungs.

Crash dieting and constant fluctuations in weight can be just as harmful as being over-weight. Hence, it is better to take a long-term approach to weight control than loosing too much too quickly. One of the best ways to improve the health of the heart is to keep blood pressure within healthy limits. Poor fitness, being overweight, eating too much salt are some of the reasons for high blood pressure. The higher the blood pressure, the harder the heart has to pump making it work harder.

A wide range of foods are good for the heart, so there is ample scope for a variety of meal for the whole family, to enjoy. Base your meals around complex carbohydrate foods such as whole grain bread, pasta, rice, cereals and potatoes. These foods will ensure that even the hungriest members of the family feel satisfied and have less need for high calorie, fatty dishes. Eat generous amounts of fruit and vegetables. You can happily graze on fruit in between meals without feeling guilty. Packed with antioxidants and fibre, fruit positively protects the heart.

The key to looking after your heart and circulation is simple. You do no have to cut out your favourite food, simply moderate your intake of the foods that are less good for you and fill up on many delicious foods that protect your heart. Add to that a little extra regular physical activity and you will see your health improve dramatically.

Respiratory System

Our respiratory system is a sophisticated machine designed to extract oxygen from air and deliver it to the blood stream. Fruit and vegetables are best allies in fighting respiratory infections and maintaining healthy lungs.

Vitamin C helps to fight bacteria that cause some respiratory illnesses and Vitamin E another powerful antioxidant has a major role in the health of your lungs. Vitamin A, yet another oxidant is vital for repair of cells, especially those forming mucus lining of the lungs.

Magnesium has a direct action on respiratory health. It helps to relax the muscles of the airways. People who lack magnesium are more likely to have difficulty with their breathing than those who have high levels of it. Zinc shortens the length of time that cold lasts.

Intake of too much salt has adverse effect on the respiratory system, as too much salt makes the airways contract, thereby restricting the flow of oxygen to the lungs

Traditional remedies for respiratory illnesses - Garlic, onion and other members of the alum family are especially rich in antiviral substances. Garlic is another stimulant used to loosen the phlegm so that it can be expelled by coughing, thereby relieving congested airways. Live yogurt is also very helpful to boost immunity towards respiratory illnesses.

Last but not the least, cigarette smoking - Cigarette smoking is very destructive to the lungs and immune system. The damage is done whether one inhales the smoke directly or through passive smoking. Giving up smoking is one of the best things one can do to protect one's health. Smoking causes serious long-term damage, leading to cancer, heart disease, strokes and rheumatoid arthritis.

Some foods are richer than others in important nutrients that help protect our respiratory. It can be got from the following sources:

Vitamin C

Fresh fruit and vegetables, and fruit juices are rich in Vitamin C.

Vitamin A

Fish oils, dairy products, spinach, liver, carrots, apricots and margarine.

Vitamin E

Seed oils such as corn oil, sunflower oil, outer germ of cereals, olive oil, pears, avocados, muesli, nuts, green leafy vegetables, whole wheat bread, cereals and egg yolks.

Beta carotene

Orange, red, yellow and dark green fruit and vegetables such as carrots, red peppers, spinach, mangoes, peaches and apricots.

Magnesium

Naturally present in refined cereals and vegetables, peanuts and wholemeal bread.

Zinc

Lean red meat, liver, shell fish (especially oysters), egg yolks, whole grain cereals and pulses.

Digestive System

A good digestive system is the cornerstone of one's health. Yet, we observe that many people take for granted this system, and only awaken when something goes wrong. Choosing the right foods is the best way to ensure that the digestive system functions at its best and one gets the maximum benefit out of it.

"A bad digestion is the root of all evil"
- Hippocrates, 400 BC

Our supply of nutrients depends upon not just the food we eat but also on how we digest and absorb it. Hence, proper chewing the food before we swallow it is of immense value. Each morsel is broken down by the teeth and mixed with the saliva. The saliva contains enzymes which begin the breakdown of starch into nutrients, that can be eventually be absorbed across the gut and into the blood stream.

More and more people are actively pursuing a healthy lifestyle. Take charge of your health. The food you eat affects every part of your body. Healthy skin and shiny hair are the immediate signs, that you are getting the right nutrients and also an accurate reflection of your state of health. It makes all the difference to your energy levels, your resistance to infection, alertness, strength and endurance. With a well-balanced diet you can build foundations for your long-term well-being.

The supportive framework for your body, the skeleton is made of bones. Working in harmony with your muscles and aided by joints, bones enable you to move around and help to protect your internal organs. Building and maintaining healthy bones play a major role in keeping you mobile and flexible. The best approach to maintaining strong bones through life is to follow a healthy lifestyle with a balanced diet and regular exercise.

Food restriction in any form, such as elimination diets and wellness diets are said to upset hormonal regulation, partially setting off serious mental and physical health problem and paradoxically gain weight instead of weight loss.

Do you want to enter the sixth or seventh decade of your life without obesity, hypertension, coronary heart disease and diabetes?

- ✓ Cut out or cut down the white devils such as pasta, white bread, polished rice and potatoes. It will help you to lose weight and have tons of energy
- ✓ Eat good levels of protein. Excess though, will accumulate fat. Lean piece of fish or chicken with each meal can give plenty of protein
- ✓ Eat leafy dark green vegetables. They help to beat osteoporosis, a common phenomenon seen these days
- ✓ It takes tremendous amount of energy to digest our food. When we fill our stomach with foods, that are harder to digest, such as meat, more of our body resources are called in to aid the digestive process. These foods, though give you a quick spike of energy. However, later a sudden

feeling of lethargy creeps in. Have you ever noticed after a heavy meal; you feel sleepy and lethargic?

✓ Eat plenty of vegetables and fruits, they take a lot less energy to digest

✓ Carbonated drinks can be replaced with fresh juices or some nice mineral water. It will save you from extra calories and above all save your life. I have seen the adverse effect of the carbonated drinks, has had on one of my nephews. Belonging to an affluent class, he was conditioned to drink a cola to quench his thirst. Water was a big "No-No". This continued for years at a stretch. After some years, he developed some breathing problem. On consulting the doctor, he was advised to stop drinking any carbonated drink and start drinking water.

✓ Stay away from refined sugar, it isn't energy efficient

Our approach should be, *"There's only one life, so enjoy food, eat better, exercise regularly, sleep well and walk through a great, amazing journey of life".*

Chapter Two

Healthy Mind in a Healthy Body

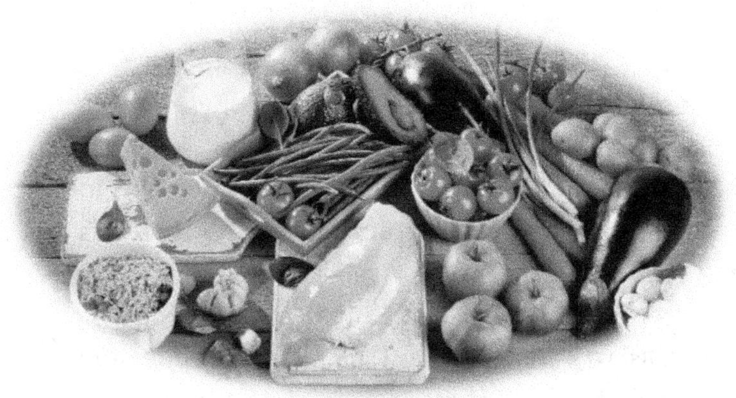

"You can either suffer the pain of discipline or the pain of regret"

-Jim Rohn

Some key rules to set on the journey to "Healthy mind and a Healthy body"

Self-discipline

Self-discipline has always proved as a key element for success in field of our life. Naturally, health being a part of overall success, if governed by some rules will go a long way in progressing and maintaining good health.

Moderation the golden rule

"If we could give every individual the right amount of nourishment and exercise, not too little and not too much, we would have found the safest way to health"
                                        -Hippocrates

Food consumed in moderation will keep our physiological system in order, at the same time help us enjoy variety of food throughout our life. Over indulgence may result in illness, which may not permit you to have certain foods which may add to the intensity of the illness. It, therefore, is in our interest to eat in moderation and continue to enjoy and relish a variety of food, at the same time stay healthy and fit. Moderation is a relative term, considering we all are of different sizes and shape. Moderation for a tall healthy person may be excessive for a medium size person, so on and so forth. In view of this "one size fits all" formula does not apply here. One thing is clear, our body gives us signals as to our food needs. The closer our chemistry with our body, the better we will understand it.

Further, we have heard this saying from times immemorial and practised by a number of centenarians **"Eat less, live longer"**. Studies reveal that a number of centenarians have lived a healthy active life eating light, minimal meals. They ate to live and not lived to eat. Living at a tolerable level of hunger, before you eat means that you are eating to refuel, not for entertainment, out of habit or for emotional fulfilment. However, the times have changed, life styles have become lavish, incomes have topped the roof and so our eating habits. We indulge in rich and abundant food. Though, I am not in a position to advocate any principle, I myself feel a balance between the two, will help us have the best of both the worlds.

Habits make you what you are

"We are what we repeatedly do. Excellence then is not an act but a habit"

-Aristotle

"Motivation is what gets you started. Habits is what keeps you going"

-Jim Ryin

We all are governed by our habits, which are created by us and only us. Our food habits are normally picked up during our childhood from our parents. What you eat, how you eat, and when you eat all has a tremendous effect on your health. It has been taught to all of us that we should eat our food slowly, enjoying every morsel chewing it thoroughly to get the best from it. However, today's busy life gives us no option, but to have our meals in the time available, which has become a rare commodity today. Over the last few decades, the meal eating patterns have changed from substantial breakfasts, main meals at midday and light dinners to light quick breakfasts, snack lunches and main meal, eaten either on return from work or even late nights. The heavy meals in the evening or night, encourages more food energy to be converted into fats, the reason being, we relax and do not exercise after the meal. This lifestyle has a heavy toll on our health. Being over-weight has become a common phenomenon. Some minor changes in these habits can go a long way towards attaining good health on a consistent basis.

We have been hearing since a very long time, "Have breakfast like a king, lunch like a common man and dinner like a pauper" to live a long and healthy life. However, how many of us apply this to our life? A negligible few. I still remember, during my working days in Mumbai, there was a senior official, who was tall, healthy and fit. We used to travel to work in the same contract bus, so would have some great discussions on topics that would add value to our thinking. One day, I asked him about the secret of his health, to which he did reply but first questioned me, "what made me ask such a question, when I was fit and fine" Those days, I was in the peak of my health. He said "No secret, just I have my meals at regular times irrespective of the place I am". He started his day with a full meal, lunch would be simple with a fruit and most importantly had an early dinner. A glass of warm milk before going to bed. What discipline! But the main secret of his good health lay in the intake of food in moderation. So rightly it is said, anything in moderation is good and in excess is harmful.

A diet plan can be designed, taking into consideration the pattern of foods we are used to, culture, religion, geographical situation, so on and so forth. The golden rule, however, that can be followed, is to plan a diet in such a way that you receive all the necessary nutrients and to add some appeal put in some variety to it. When it comes to health, the common saying "An apple a day keeps the doctor away" keeps on coming off and on. I totally agree with it. I have been eating an apple daily since I remember. It was always a part of my lunch. Fruits and vegetables have been an important part of my daily meals, though I am a non-vegetarian. As I mentioned before, in today's rush times, it has become near to impossible to have an elaborate breakfast. The same situation, I had gone through some years back, when I was staying alone, because of my transfer to a new place. I, then found an innovative way to start my day with good nutrition. I would pack a bowl of cornflakes with some cold milk to which I would add plenty of dry fruits such as almonds, some dry fig, dates, cashews, raisins and add some natural honey for sweetness. Trust me this bowl of magic ingredients kept me energetic throughout the day. On returning from work, I would just have 2 healthy biscuits and go for my work out to the gym without any rest. This was the level of energy this wonderful breakfast gave me. So, you see we can and are capable of creating some innovative dishes to suit our lifestyle and at the same time have a great day, a day of energy and vitality. As long as one has a commitment to one's health.

Chapter Three

Exercise

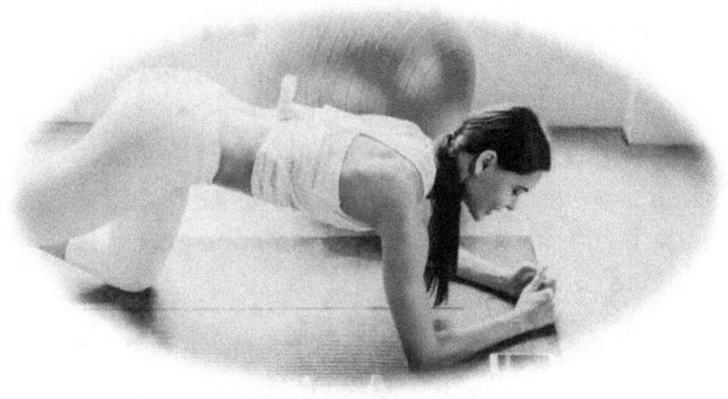

"To keep the body in good health is a duty otherwise we shall not be able to keep the mind strong and clear"
-Buddha

Exercise makes you feel better and have more energy. It's a major component of life of health and fulfilment.

Exercise is the perfect partner of a good diet, whether it be a weight-reducing one or just a healthy, balanced diet. Not only does it burn off calories, but makes the muscles firmer, redistributes the bodyweight and improves posture. With exercise not only will you look and feel healthier and sleep better, but will find that you are more energetic and alert and less prone to tension and tiredness.

Our bodies are filled with toxins from the air we breathe and from the pesticides on the food we eat. Our good health depends on moving them out of our system. That's one of the things exercises does, when you exercise the body perspires, and gets rid of the toxins. It also gets the blood and lymphatic systems pumping. The increased flow of blood is good for the brain and also lifts our mood. Exercise helps prevent many diseases, such as cancer, heart attack, heart disease, diabetes and controls blood sugar and blood pressure.

It lowers stress and promotes weight loss. In today's world of multi-tasking, we go through immense stress. Some of us do cope up mainly due to our good health, however, majority of us are pulled down to such an extent that it takes a toll on our bodies. Exercise will help us cope with this situation, at the same time give us the fulfilment of achieving all our goals, be it personal as well as professional. Along with that, exercise also improves the immune system and can fulfil a dream every one dreams of "Slowing down the aging process".

Follow the mantra ***"Move as if Your Life Depended on it - it Does"***

There are innumerable benefits we gain from Exercise. Besides the benefits stated above here are some more, though they are innumerable:

- Exercise builds strong bones
- Exercise improves digestion and promotes frequent bowel movements
- Exercise gives you restful sleep
- Exercise prevents colds and flu
- Exercise reduces depression
- Exercise refreshes your body, renews your energy and gives you strength

"True enjoyment comes from the activity of the mind and exercise of the body, the two are ever united"
-Wilhelm von Humboldt

Hopefully all these benefits should inspire one and all to give due importance to exercise. It has been observed that the persons who are dedicated to their health, their exercise routine is inspired within and hence stay committed and live by it, under any circumstances. I always enjoyed exercising and derived excitement from various activities, especially dancing, swimming, trekking and various sports. This inner happiness kept me committed from young age to some form of exercise or other, giving me an additional benefit of wonderful exposure to varied sports activities. Regular walking and playing Badminton gave an additional dose to my body, making it strong and flexible.   This passion led me to become a regular member of a health club. When anyone shifts his or her residence, they always look out for a place, where their passion can be fulfilled, be it reading, playing, dancing, singing, exercising, etc. My sister is an avid reader, books are a part of her life. She discovers a book library, where ever she resides. And as for me, I search for a health club in the vicinity of my new home.

We often hear from people of signing up for membership of a health club with great enthusiasm and dreams in their eyes. However, except for some, we come across a number of them, who are unable to keep the interest alive, as it requires self-discipline and consistency and sometimes sacrifice to come out of their comfort zone. This results in discontinuing and getting back to their earlier regular sedentary routine. Such an attitude has a two-fold effect, one slow health deterioration and second devaluation of one's own money and filling the pockets of the Health Club owners, without an inch of return for the money spent. Being a Finance and a Life coach, in my opinion money or time invested should always give you some return. And here you are just dwindling away your own money for nothing.

Exercise takes motivation and most people make the mistake of thinking they have to be motivated to start exercising, But, that's a faulty logic. Do the thing and you'll get the energy to do the thing. Start exercising and you'll get motivated, not the other way around. Lack of exercise makes one sluggish and feel exhausted, while exercise makes you feel energetic and renewed.

Another observation is that, a number of people in their late 40's and early 50's joining the Gym, with the expectation of getting into form. Most of them have as good as never exercised in their life. Great! Nice to see this new awareness of one's health. However, it's worth thinking that you have never or hardly exercised for almost 4 decades of your life and all of a sudden you expect your body to support a rigorous exercise. Excuse me, I do not mean to discourage. On the contrary, I admire and appreciate their initiative. However, there is always a way to begin anything new, and like any other activity, training in a gym also needs to start gradually, step by step. Like, if one wants to climb a mountain, he or she has to walk regularly, increasing the distance gradually, in order to develop stamina required to climb a mountain. Similarly, for a rigorous workout sheer walking, initially with gradual improvement will not only give the confidence to exercise but also help in sustaining it on a long-term basis. The body due to lack of exercise in the previous years has become pretty stiff and lacks flexibility. Hence, the body may not be able to adapt to any rigorous exercise, in the beginning. The training may require immense effort and may result in body pain, discouraging you to continue. The saying "Slow and steady wins the race" is true. Increasing your stamina and energy level slowly and steadily will help you reach your goal; you came with in mind with. "Action takers are winners", however, subject to they are on the right track and the right mode. So, stay inspired and continue exercising as per your capacity.

"The purpose of training is to tighten the slack, toughen the body and polish the spirit"
                                                    -Morihei Ueshiba

Another set of people are those who purchase exercise gadgets, seeing the ever so perfect models. In 90% of the cases, these gadgets stay unutilized and are seen lying idle either under the beds or lying somewhere in the home gathering dust. The irony is, we often see treadmills being used as a drying stand! This may be due to the initial interest just fading away due to either not much progress being seen in the initial stage or total loss of interest. In this context, we can relate to the growth of a bamboo tree. A bamboo tree takes years and years to grow beyond the ground level, however, after it shoots above the land surface it grows very high within few months. The moral behind this is that to achieve some significant result, it always takes time and patience. Patience always pays, the same applies to exercise. Be patient, be consistent and most importantly be positive. Further, people who start their exercise routine in their early years of life, always have an edge over others, as they have tuned their body for the best of their health. As the saying goes "An early bird gets the worm", so start at the earliest, start today before you miss the bus. As we all know, time just flies and we do not realise, unless something triggers and force us to take action.

Exercise should be a life-long habit. And once cultivated will become a part of our life. Regular exercise before you are 30, when the bone density is achieved, means strong bones. After this, when the bone density is lessened by the natural process of aging, continuing to get plenty of exercise helps the bones stay strong. It's therefore wise, to build an exercise routine into our schedule, say like an important Doctor's appointment. Choosing a convenient time for a workout, preferably before breakfast or lunch would be great. Though the time may differ as per one's convenience and time availability. During my working days I would go to the gym in the evening and it served me perfectly. The only caution, I took was I never had any food for at least 3 hours before the workout. Another important tip for getting the best out of the workout would be to exercise without any distraction, especially staying away from connectivity like the mobile. This will help you to concentrate fully without any distraction and enjoy your workout to the maximum. By the way, many reputed Gymnasiums and Health clubs do not allow the use of mobiles inside. A good system, as firstly, it shows their dedication to the purpose of operating a health club and secondly, setting the ethics behind the workout, a necessity for focussing on the activity.

Choice of exercise is up to the individual, his age or her age, health, lifestyle, temperament, liking and definitely the economic condition. There are innumerable ways of exercise to choose from, depending on the situation of the person, the secret however, lies in choosing one that you enjoy, so you exercise regularly. For some yoga may be ideal, if his temperament and his lifestyle suit it. For some, just a walk may be fine, for a young robust youth a vigorous aerobic dance may attract, for a teenager running or cycling may suit to her or his taste, so on and so forth. Some need motivation and company, and to their advantage there are a number of group activities such as Zumba, aerobics, dancing and even yoga. Selection of an appropriate exercise is important and without any doubt, should be enjoyable, then half the battle won.

As we grow older, our bones lose density. Applying any kind of stress to our muscles, which is what we do when we lift weights, for example, builds up bone density. Muscle mass also decreases as we age; exercise can help reclaim it. All we need is minimum thirty minutes of exercise five days a week. You use muscles every minute of the day, even just to sit on a chair or stand upright. As with bones, exercise is the best way to maintain healthy muscles. Without exercise our muscles will decrease in size and we will lose strength, suppleness and flexibility.

Have you wondered, why elderly people fall so often? It is usually because they don't have strong thigh muscles. If you work on thighs every day, just by sitting down and getting up over and over again, you will be far less likely to fall, because your legs stay strong. You can prevent the falls and broken hips, that are the number one reason why people go to nursing homes today. To build muscles, you need progressive resistance, meaning that you gradually stress your muscles more and more.

Motivation and inspiration play a key role in sustaining your interest in exercise. Unconsciously, all of us desire for good health and a beautiful toned body, however few of us are self-inspired to pursue this desire on long term. Last year, the gymnasium I was going to, advertised about a concessional medical insurance plan for members whose attendance to the gymnasium would be minimum 85 percent for a year. What a unique way to motivate people to exercise regularly. Such motivation will go a long way for the members. Most importantly they will get positive results in their health and thus stay self-motivated and self-inspired.

Various forms of Exercises

"Training gives us an outlet for suppressed energies created by stress and thus tones the spirit just as exercise conditions the body"
-Arnold Schwarzenegger

To enable to choose the appropriate form of exercise, information on various forms and their benefits are given below:

Yoga

Yoga is a means of balancing and harmonizing the body, mind and emotions. It combines low-impact exercise with stretching and breathing. Yoga is different from most of the other forms of exercise in that, it is not concerned with how many repetitions are performed or how well a person performs a particular exercise. Instead yoga focuses your attention on how your body is structured and how to move without aggravating any injury or causing pain. It teaches you to breathe properly and to integrate breathing with the positions of the body. You don't strain or force your body when doing yoga, rather it gently stretches various muscles. It improves strength, flexibility and endurance. There are several types of yoga, Hatha Yoga being popular. Power Yoga has also become popular in the recent years. It is generally preferred by athletes to develop strength and stamina.

Aerobic Exercise

Aerobic means "in the presence of air". It's a kind of exercise that gets you breathing deeply and more rapidly than normal. Aerobic exercises generally work on the large muscle groups of the body in repetitive motions for sustained period of time. Walking, jogging, cycling, skipping, swimming, dancing are all forms of aerobic exercises.

Walking

Walking is the simplest way to improve health. Walking improves the circulation, stimulates the heart and lungs, loosens the joints and helps walker lose weight. Walking does not involve any violent exertion and hence has no side effects. On the contrary, it has the advantage of being something that can be done every day, and by almost anyone, regardless of age and state of health. If you have not been walking regularly and need company, get a partner and start walking. You may start slowly and gradually increase the time till you reach at least 30 minutes per day. It will not only energise you but help you to keep your weight in control and above all give you a new confidence raising your self-esteem. Brisk walking is one of the best forms of exercise. It can give you three times the normal amount of oxygen you would otherwise get. I had read somewhere years back, before you start walking especially in a natural environment, take a deep breath when you start walking. This helps in inhaling maximum oxygen in each breath while walking. One caution that needs to be taken, is while walking a good pair of shoes is a must. It will not injure your feet. And a soft walking surface also matters, as hard and especially uneven surface can injure the joints. This experience I have had. When I was in Mumbai, I always walked on a jogging track. However, when I was posted to Bhopal, I would walk daily for a minimum an hour or even more in the colony compound which was hard and uneven. After eight years of walking my knees started giving me pain, there was wear and tear of my knee bones and hence had to go through knee replacement. Touch wood, today I am fine and continue to exercise and walk normally and have even climbed the Tiger's nest. Thanks to my consistent exercise routine.

Jogging

Jogging an excellent for heart, lungs and circulation. The more you jog, the more you burn calories and stronger your muscles become. Almost anyone of any age can jog safely, even if your health is poor, provided your doctor approves of it. You do not have to achieve any particular speed, nor is it necessary to jog every day. Building up stamina you may gradually jog for 15 minutes three times a week, more if you can manage it.

Running

Running is an excellent all-round exercise for the heart and lungs, muscle strength and endurance. Running is only for the fit and healthy. It is generally unsuitable for anyone over the age of 40, unless they have been running since their younger days or else, they need to prepare for it with another sport or regular jogging. To build up slowly to the goal set, begin with a mixture of jogging, running and walking to avoid strain on the muscles and heart.

Skipping

Skipping can form a part of body-building programme, to strengthen the muscles or it can be used to shape figure, by tightening the muscles and loose flesh, making the thighs and calves firmer and shapely and improve posture. Either way, skipping is a good warm-up activity, promotes stamina and coordination and is a good exercise for the heart and lungs. And the best part of it, is that it requires a small investment of a skipping rope with your time. Aim to build up to 15 minutes a day.

Cycling

Cycling is an excellent aerobic exercise for the legs, for the heart and for the lungs. Age, arthritis, heart or lung conditions, including asthma, are no bar to cycling, providing you have first consulted your doctor.

Swimming

Swimming is a wonderful and safe way to exercise, as water provides support, so you do not strain any part of your body. This is particularly useful when you are overweight. Thirty minutes of sustained swimming a day increases your stamina, suppleness and strength. It also tones your body and who does not like a well-toned body. Elderly people with arthritis problems are advised to walk in water. In the recent years, water aerobics have become a very popular and enjoyable sport. Here I would like to share my experience on scuba diving. A few years back I was in Andaman & Nicobar to celebrate my birthday. As mentioned before, I try something new on my birthdays. This birthday, I ventured into scuba diving. To my surprise despite having those heavy oxygen cylinders on my back, when I went deep the waters, I became totally light and weightless. This is the effect water has on our weight. A beautiful experience, gliding effortlessly within the waters enjoying the sights of colourful fish, a treat to watch and the best gift for my birthday.

Badminton

Badminton is an indoor game, which promotes suppleness throughout the body and builds up powers of endurance. Played vigorously, badminton is a fine exercise for the heart and lungs. As an overhead game, it is especially good for strengthening the back and shoulders and improving posture. Although it is strenuous at a high level, you can enjoy a more social game without over-exertion, particularly mixed doubles. Provided you are reasonably fit, you can take up badminton well into middle age.

Squash

Squash is the fastest game on two legs. Playing for about 30 to 45 minutes will help lose weight, make you more supple, faster on your feet and improve your staying power. Being an indoor game, it can be played throughout the year.

Table tennis

You are interested in a muscular body; this is the game to be played with full body exertion. However, on a lesser level the game exercises the lungs and heart, gets you on your toes and improves coordination.

Tennis

A hard game of singles burns up calories, exercises the heart and lungs, increases suppleness and helps in tightening of stomach muscles in particular and can be still fun. A gentle game of mixed doubles tennis is fun along with the exercising your entire body.

Dance

All forms of dancing are an excellent exercise and most importantly enjoyable. They aid coordination, flexibility, and suppleness. Dance is good for the heart and lungs and if done energetically, will even help reduce weight. There are several forms of dance to choose from, such as Indian classical dance, folk dance, western dance, ballroom dance, modern dance, and so on.

Calisthenics

Callisthenics is getting weight training benefits by using your own body to build muscles. It includes push-ups, pull-ups, sit-ups, lungs, calf raises and many more. You can do these without any equipment. Weight training and callisthenics are a part of a holistic approach to exercise plus they build strong bones and muscles. Stretching promotes flexibility and can serve as a good warm-up prior to exercise.

Pilates

Pilates is a form of exercise, which has become popular in the recent years. It consists of precise movements requiring control and form. It emphasises on proper alignment, centring, concentration, breathing and flowing movements.

Tai Chi

Tai Chi is an ancient Chinese form of meditation expressed through slow, graceful and dance-like movement. It involves and benefits the mind and the body. It involves slow smooth movements with rhythmic abdominal breathing. It's great for older people, especially those who suffer from arthritis. Tai Chi movements help improve muscle mass, strength, stamina, balance, coordination, flexibility and tones muscles. In China, regular exercise starts early. The children are taught Tai Chi. This art, however, can be learned from a trained instructor.

Regular stretching before and after exercise keeps you flexible, allowing you to move more freely and feel more at ease with your body.

Rest a rejuvenation exercise of life

Sleep

Good sleep is one of the best principles for good health, yet relatively few people get adequate sleep. Our addiction to the digital world, makes us cheat on our sleep requirement. It has been advised by several doctors having regular time for sleeping helps us sleep well and rejuvenate our bodies. Yet, in the today's hectic world, it is observed sleep deprivation has become a norm of the day. Less sleep increases one's chances to suffer from heart attack, stroke, diabetes, weight gain and premature aging. It is said that an average adult needs seven to nine hours of sleep. It's not just the length of sleep that is important. The quality of sleep also matters and makes a difference in the quality of life one leads. Middle aged and elderly people sleep less than the younger people

Are you getting enough sleep?

There are certain indications that you are not getting adequate sleep, such as inability to wake up without an alarm, feeling drowsy during the day, waking up feeling irritated and crappy and waking up with a slightest sound. Stress and anxiety are number one reason for insomnia. Insomnia has many causes and patterns, however some common causes are smoking and drinking alcohol, eating high sugar foods before sleep and having cups of coffee, chocolate and soft drinks. Alcohol is thought by many to be a good sleep inducer. It may send you off to sleep for short time, but as the alcohol is absorbed into the blood, it acts as a stimulant that wakes you up, and sends your mind active and racing. As a result, you cannot get back to sleep again. Even vigorous exercise few hours before going to bed may interfere with your sleep. The person who cannot get off to sleep is usually tense, insecure or anxious of something. The most common emotion that stops people sleeping is resentment, if you feel you have been treated unfairly. You may lie for hours thinking about it.

A good night's sleep restores, repairs and rejuvenates your body. It also improves the immune system of the body along with slowing down the aging process. It is said preparing for sleep in the night begins during daytime.

Below are few things that can improve your chances of having a good and comfortable night's sleep:

1. Daily exercise
2. Eating moderate healthy meals, especially eating a light meal at least four hours before going to bed induces good quality sleep.
3. Maintaining a bedtime ritual and relaxation of the body and mind before going to bed ensures good sound sleep.
4. Make sure your bedroom is well-ventilated and is comfortable for you, neither too cold or too hot.
5. Invest in the best mattress you can afford. If you are uncomfortable, you will not be able to sleep well.
6. Wear comfortable loose clothes.
7. Take a warm drink at bedtime, a milky one rather than tea or coffee, Though I know of people who sleep well even after drinking hot tea. So, it's up to you and your system.
8. Have a warm water bath. It works in a similar way as a warm drink.
9. Try to do something relaxing before you go to bed. It depends on you, some find reading a book relaxing, some may find watching their favourite show on TV relaxing, etc. Finally, the objective to relax and keep away from unwanted thoughts.

Following healthy sleeping habits will keep at bay insomnia and any other illnesses related to sleep deprivation.

Oxygen – Breathing exercise

Oxygen is the most important nutrient in the body. You can go weeks without food, days without water, but only minutes without oxygen. Most people oxygenate their system poorly. All traditions have their breathing practices, as breath is life.

The ancients would start their day with deep diaphragmatic breathing.

Most adults breathe high and in their chest. When breathing properly, deep from the diaphragm, your abdomen should extend, this isn't popular with a population that spends a lot of energy sucking it in. If you want to see a great example of how to breathe, watch a small baby. When a baby breathes, its stomach extends.

Deep breathing energises and heals us.

Take long, slow breathes, inhaling deeply through the nose, then exhaling fully from the diaphragm, to eliminate toxins and stress.

There are several different ways to breathe, but in your normal daily activities, healthy neutral breathing consists of 1:1 ratio of breathing in and out is good. So, for instance, if you breathe in four counts you would like-wise breathe out for four.

Make it a part of your day to practise conscious deep diaphragmatic breathing and very soon it will become a habit, that you will no longer have to think about. You may be surprised to see, how much energy you will have. Next time, you feel tired instead of going for some drink, try some deep breaths and observe the total shift of your energy. This technique is very effective and much healthier. Proper breathing is one of the best ongoing relaxation and de-stressing technique.

Building an exercise program

"Take care of your body. It's the only place you have to live"

-Jim Rohn

Building an exercise program into your schedule doesn't have to be boring; it can be as fun as you make it. Find exercises that you enjoy doing, such as swimming, dancing, may be playing a game of badminton or tennis etc. In addition to this you can look for opportunities to fit in activities, that will enhance your health and vitality, such as gardening, parking your vehicle in a space farthest away from your office or a store, take steps instead of the elevator and so on. I remember the days, when I would climb up and down   seven floors to my office some years back. There was a middle-aged officer, who never used the elevator to climb up the seven floors to the office. I was thoroughly impressed with his energy, strength and vitality and most importantly his climbing the seven floors. One fine day I asked him about it, he said why don't you try smilingly. I did try the very next day and was highly surprised to see it was effortless. Since then, I never used the elevator to the office, irrespective of the number of times I had to during the day.

Like water, when our bodies are stagnant, they breed disease. It's time to stir the waters of your life and start exercising.

Rethink and redesign your schedule to squeeze in some movement on a daily basis. Getting the form is important. Design an exercise workout as per your need, taking into various considerations various aspects, such as your body dimensions, time availability and most importantly the resources available. Set your goals for the type of the exercise you will be doing. Start slowly, gradually increase and reach the desired level, you feel is right for you. The reason, being everyone is unique; everyone is different so do not go by other's standards. Set your own standard. Our body gives us signals to know our limits. Choosing an exercise location is also very important. Some people jog by the side of the road, where vehicles move pumping out petrol and diesel exhaust. Eat fresh homemade, seasonal food on time and in moderation. Get enough sleep.

A fit body harbours a fit and healthy mind. People are making time for functional fitness, such as swimming, cycling, jogging and running that keeps them fit and close to nature. Awareness that you are doing something good and positive for your bone density, cardio-vascular health and cognitive abilities, every single time you exercise can add to the good feelings that makes exercise easier to sustain. Ultimately, feeling good on a sustainable basis, will keep you motivated and inspire you to stay healthy and fit.

Look fit and feel fit

Weight watchers are dime a dozen. They may go to any extent to fit into a gown for a bachelorette party or a tuxedo for their friend's wedding. Looking fit is not enough, feeling fit is equally important. Many of us compare our bodies with others, this means we are not appreciating our bodies, our temples, and most importantly not honouring them. Self-appreciation expands our perception of our own bodies, resulting in high self-esteem and most importantly self-confidence. Just remembered, the day of our farewell in school, the day when we were given some parting advice for our coming life in college. One particular advice which my sixth sense said was the most important was, "Do not ape anyone, be yourself". I have followed it since then and consciously developed a unique style of mine in every aspect of my life. This golden mantra has helped me live a life of high self-esteem, self-respect and self-pride. These days we hear very often from the experts of success, saying be authentic in everything you do for lasting success. Wasn't I taught the same thing in school almost 5 decades back?

A healthy mind in a healthy body

Flexible body, Flexible Mind

An inflexible body is a reflection of an inflexible mind. On a physical level, it is crucial to stay mobile and fluid. Ask yourself this, when you wake up in the morning and you feel uneasy and painful, maybe in your back or knees or neck, do you feel young or old.

It's a good idea to learn postures to stretch your shoulders and chest, hips, lower back, hamstrings and thighs on a daily basis. What's the first thing a dog or cat does after getting up from a nap? Stretch! Your exercise routine should include stretching to maintain a flexible and a supple body.

There's wisdom in listening to your body and taking time to rest when you need it.

Age – Just a number

Today aging is not getting old. People are staying fitter, feeling better and living longer then even before. Although genes play a role in the aging process, the food you eat at this time of life can make the difference to your retirement years. To get the most out of each day, you need to be fit and healthy. Staying active and eating really well will ensure life of vitality and zest for a lifetime. At this time of your life, your body becomes less efficient at absorbing and using several vitamins and minerals. You may find your appetite decreasing, however, the need for vitamins and minerals stays the same. It is, therefore, necessary to eat good nutritious food. Being overweight may increase the risk of serious illnesses such as diabetes, heart disease, etc. Hence, it is advisable to keep control of one's weight. It can also put extra pressure on the joints, giving pain to the joints or even can result in arthritis. Try to get around 30 minutes of continuous exercise every day, go for a walk, do some gardening, enjoy some pleasurable active pastime. Finally, the most important thing to remember, is that age is just a number. It's you who is a reflection of your age. Positive attitude and living in the moment, will keep you enjoying every moment of your life.

A number of successful senior citizens are living a happy, fulfilling life and most importantly an active life full of energy and vitality. Some living examples are Warren Buffet, Bill Gates, Richard Branson, Mukesh Ambani,

Oprah Winfrey, Robert Kiyosaki and many more. All of them are unstoppable, driven with optimum energy and zest for life. They are living with a strong purpose in life and above all are inclined to contribute to the world the best of themselves.

Chapter Four

Take Charge of your precious body

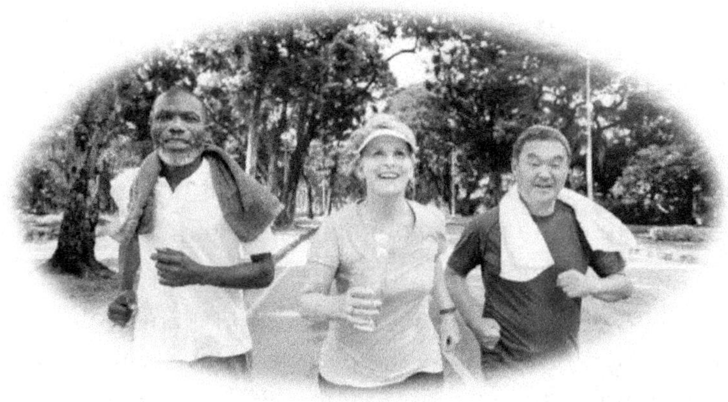

"It is health that's real wealth, and not pieces of gold and silver"

-Mahatma Gandhi

We were born with greatness, but sadly get conditioned into mediocrity over time. We all can be healthy, strong and fit with what the Creator has given us to work with. Various religious traditions call the human form the precious Human body or the Temple. What are you putting into your temple? Do you treat it so that, it will easily and elegantly carry you through a long and fulfilling life? Or do you stuff it with junk to satisfy your short-term desires? How do you move your temple through the world? Have you ever thought about the fact, it takes a few minutes of your time, an investment in yourself to walk a couple of flights up instead of taking an elevator? Remember, I mentioned before about climbing seven floors to my office? It truly gave me a sense of achievement, every time I climbed.

In order for you to treat yourself as a priceless artefact that you are, you've got to see yourself as such.

Everyone has been gifted with wonderful qualities and one of them is the physical quality. It is said, things that are appreciated increase in value and when you are grateful for it, you are saying to the Universe, "Thank you and give me more". Some people are in love with being out of shape, as they are attending to it all the time. "Oh! I am busy, I just do not have the time to exercise", "My kids keep me fully occupied, leaving no time for myself", so on and so forth.

Further, every single time, you look in the mirror and say something derogatory about your body, you are being in love with that out of form body. This self-talk results in self-sabotage. Such people wonder "How is it that some of the people stay in good shape and do not put on extra weight". They do not realise, they too can have a beautifully shaped body, its just that they need to make a key shift in their mindset. As you shift mentally, emotionally and physically, your image in the mirror begin to morph and reflect what you think and feel.

Start asking "What I love about my body", "What do I appreciate about my body?". Think deep, you will observe a number of things about your body that are good which deserve appreciation and for which you should be grateful for. As you love and appreciate and are grateful for who you are and what you are, then you begin to take different care of yourself. You start noticing your plus points and may even notice that certain parts of your body, for example the waistline or stomach, if attended to may get into a better shape. This awareness will inspire you to work on your body with sincerity and dedication. As is known, "Energy flows where attention goes", stay focussed on the positive and not the negative.

To stay focused, it is a known fact that affirmations can help us to a great extent. Fortunately, for me affirmations have helped me tremendously. They keep me in align with my desired outcomes. For health, I have been using the following two affirmations:

"The gift of health is keeping me alive"

"I am becoming stronger, more vital and youthful everyday"

Imagine, you were given an Aladdin's lamp and could have the body and health of your dreams, what would it look like?

Imagine how it would feel to go clothes shopping and find that everything fits in your dream size?

How rewarding would it be to be fit older adult with a perfect or almost perfect figure?

These questions will give clarity on the sort of person you would love to be seen as. The picture will help you to kick start with your journey towards a new you.

Invest your time in the activities worthy of who you are and who you want to become. Its your precious body, your temple. Treat it that way.

One secret of consistent energy lies in eating little and often, and eating energy-filled foods, as close to their natural state as possible, rather than sugar-laden snacks.

A high-performance body is like a high-performance vehicle. Its high maintenance vehicle that gives you high performance. The more evolved and high performance you choose to become, the more effort you will have to put into maintaining a high level of health, fitness and vitality.

When we talk about physical part of our body, we equate it with the tangible. We choose the food we eat; we choose the exercise we indulge in, therein feeling our body muscles exercise, tone and rebuild the temple of our bodies. However, beyond this, there is an invisible intangible foundation of thoughts and words, which have an immense effect on the physical part of our body. Many people have a physical weakness or two or three, such as neck pain, back pain or maybe a sensitive stomach. We talk about it quite often, giving us the negative energy.

Your overall health has much to do about it, are you loving yourself and your life? Or are you loving your illness? Are you empowered with such negative thinking? Naturally not. You need to understand that your words, your feelings, your language can harm you. Words make your your world. Words and your feelings make your beliefs and your body obeys your beliefs.

In view of the above, a shift in your thinking, your language is needed to receive the fruits of your efforts towards good health. As Jim Rohn says "For things to change, you have to change". Energy goes where focus lies. Hence, a new shift will eliminate weakness to a great extent and achieve the desired outcomes. It's like living in the light ignoring the dark. Affirmations help in carrying out a radical shift in our thinking.

As you go through your day, get into the habit of checking in yourself regularly and asking yourself the following questions:

Does this activity fit in with my goals?

Is this food or drink going to strengthen me or not?

Are my habits in alignment with my intentions and goals?

Am I spending or investing time?

Am I contributing to self-care today?

Are my thoughts focused on the end result?

Answers to these questions will give an indication of whether you are on the right track to good health.

In case, you are someone, who believes that we have God within us and that everything happens for a reason, then isn't everything spiritual. So, pursue all your goals with equal enthusiasm, knowing that they're spiritual and believe that God, your higher self, the Universe always and only says "Yes".

Reframe your Mind

Reframing is learning to see the past, present and future in a positive light and shifting your focus away from the present point of view in order to see another person or a situation from a new perspective. Every thought you have has a ripple effect on our physical body and emotions. Thoughts lead to decisions. **It is said "the distance between the thoughts and decision is just a few seconds"**. Thus, it is very clear that thoughts play a crucial role in our life. Positive thoughts guide us to a better life, whereas negative thoughts hijack our happiness, our growth. The bad part of negative thoughts is that, it puts you in an auto-pilot mode, taking you to the past, the negative aspect time and time again.

In view of this, training our mind to focus on the positive and ignoring the negative, will go a long way to condition our mind for our betterment. Think good, positive things. **Remember the old adage, "Accentuate the positive,**

eliminate the negative". There are ways and means to stay on the positive side of life, a little difficult, however, not impossible.

- Power breathing techniques (abdominal breathing) helps to destress.
- Learning to say "No". Do not volunteer or take more activities than you are capable of handling.
- Limit the time spent with people who are pessimists, whiners or complainers (Naysayers). If you are not careful, they will drain the energy and life right out of you.
- Surround yourself with positive friends.
- Words, thoughts and attitudes are contagious, so choose friends selectively.
- Life-suckers are people who always sing the "Blame song". With life-suckers you always encourage them, whereas they always discourage you.
- If you spend a lot of time with negative people, you may land up acquiring some of their characteristics.
- It may not be possible to avoid some people, though negative. In such cases, do not let their negative attitude drain your energy, joy and strength.

Develop a positive style of life

Believe in yourself and your power to succeed. Take good care of your mind and body. Exercise, eat right and don't smoke. Optimism and living to the fullest have a rejuvenating effect on both your body and mind. It promotes good health and increases longevity. However, merely living longer does not guarantee a better life. Most of us would prefer a brief life span with quality to a long life without it. Avoid any negative entanglements that could thwart your growth. Negative emotions, such as anger, worry, resentment, anxiety, etc. lead to negative stress and make you susceptible to disease. Negative stress is corrosive energy, that has a wear-and-tear effect on both body and mind It accelerates aging and shortens our lives.

Whatever is your present age, you can control the deterioration of aging, so that your body does not self-destruct. You have the potential to live a quality, long life. Develop constructive positive energy, through healthy habits and healthy lifestyle that will empower both your body and mind. Rejuvenation plays a key role in our life, if we want to embark on the journey of younger, longer and better life. In this context, in the recent years a number health retreats have been opened for rejuvenation. It has become a part of life for several elite people. They visit the retreats for rejuvenation, relaxation and detoxification. By the way, detoxification, is a process wherein the toxins from our body are removed.

Everything starts with a purpose in mind. A purpose strong enough to wake you up with enthusiasm, a purpose to look forward to the day, weeks, months and years to come. Finding one's purpose is like half the battle one. Each one of us have some desires, desire of the life we wish to lead, desire to create a name for oneself, desire to stay healthy, wealthy and wise, so on and so forth. A purpose, therefore, is the starting point of our life's contribution to the world, our contribution to our creator and last but not the least make a difference to the society at large. All known successful people, present and past live and lived with a strong purpose in life. Take Mahatma Gandhi, his purpose was to free India from the British rule, he lived by it every second of his life and finally achieved it. We all have a purpose in life, it is intrinsic within us. All it needs is, it's discovery. Once discovered, it will give a meaning to our life and most importantly will inspire us to look after our health to fulfil that purpose.

Fit as a Fiddle Happy as a Lark

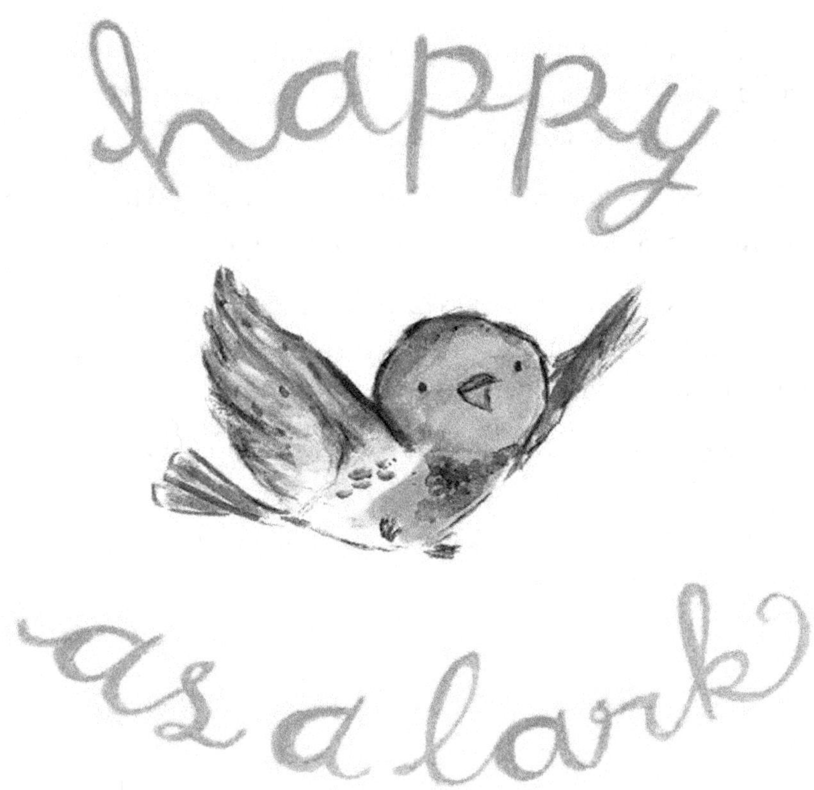

Sreeti A Amonkar

Dedication

Dedicated to my grandmother, Late Smt. Vatsalabai Laxmanshet Amonkar, who raised me to the best of her abilities despite of sort of constraints.

To my aunt, Mrs Kusum Kharangate Ramaswamy, who supported me and sheltered me in my worst days.

To, the Sonawane Family, Prakash Dada, Krushna Tai, Priyanka and Prashant, for making me a part of their family and giving me a home away from home.

And most of all to my fur-baby, Butsu, for forcing me to take a break and chill when I got too immersed in my work and thus, taking care of my emotional and physical fitness.

Introduction

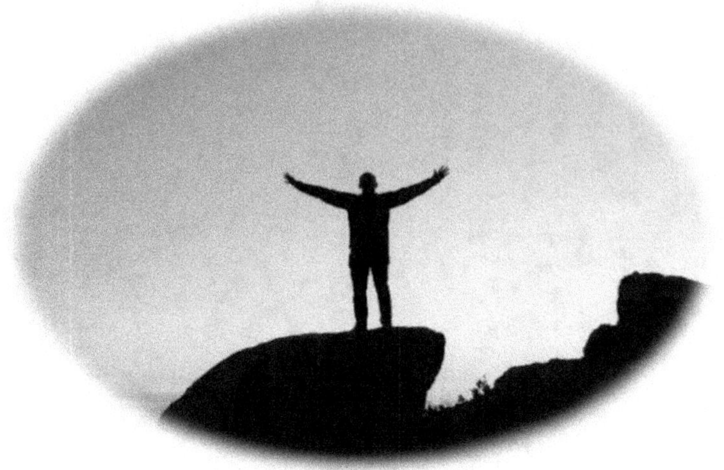

"Happiness is not something readymade. It comes from your own actions."

-Dalai Lama XIV

In my opinion, Happiness is what makes the world go round. Some might disagree and say that it's money which does it. However, the very reason why people try to amass money is that they think that it will buy the security, power, luxury, pleasure, and comfort. In today's world, money and the things money can buy, tangible like material possessions and intangible like financial security, power, etc. has turned out to be our substitute for happiness due to our ignorance even though, times and again it's been proved that money can't buy us happiness. It can only buy things that give us temporary pleasure. This feeling of pleasure which is mistaken for happiness is very shallow and transitory. Such a misconception is common and widespread. Fortuitously at the same time, more and more people have started to realise that happiness is something else and have set out on a journey that has led them inwards.

I embarked on a similar journey a couple of decades ago. The backdrop of this pursuit arose out of profound unhappiness and very dangerous levels of stress. As a child, I was abandoned by my mother and neglected by my father. I was raised by relatives who outrightly hated me and thought of me as a burden.

When I grew up, I thought of taking things in my hands. Still a teenager I had no clue what I was going to do to find an escape from my miserable life. But, one thing was for certain that I was parched for happiness and that this thirst took me on an unchartered journey. My quest for happiness forced me to go from pillar to post. From joining a far-leftist student organisation, which was needless to say, atheist, to visiting several ashrams, following spiritual gurus, and practising various paths and cults. Of course, all of these helped me in one way or the other. One thing that I got out of this in quest of mine is that there was a drastic paradigm shift in the way I perceived happiness. At least, I understood what happiness was not.

I understood that happiness, is contagious and hence with our attitude and behaviour we can make ourselves and others either happy or miserable. This insight that I got from all my years of pursuing happiness has made me believe, in sharing my happiness with whoever comes in contact with me on the journey of my life.

Our pursuit of happiness in life is very much resembling the story of 'Kasturi Mrig', the musk deer. The deer keeps wandering in the forest in search of a sweet fragrance. It is beguiled and enthralled, wondering where is the source of this enchanting smell coming from? And is unknown to the fact that the smell so inviting is possessed by its own body, right under its belly button. It's a fallacy with which it spends its lifetime, unaware of the truth.

Aren't we humans having a much similar illusion about happiness? Why are we searching for it everywhere in the world, when we can find it within, within our innate self? When are we going to shift our paradigm about happiness and set ourselves free from the shackles of misconceptions?

Finding answers to such questions will need patience. Finding your real self and your purpose of existence will need persistence. Finding happiness in its real form will need perseverance. Together, with patience, persistence, and perseverance, you will experience pure bliss. **You will be free from all negativity and become one with true happiness. And this pursuit of happiness will bring peace. Peace within and everywhere in the world.**

Imagine a world where every single human understands the fact that happiness is not something extrinsic. It is to be felt within and not without. By within, I mean inside yourself and in every moment. It may be momentary or may last for a lifetime, but it remains inside you. Happiness is immaterial of worldly things. You need not be a millionaire to be happy; you just need to feel it without greed, without arrogance, without ignorance. Once this thought takes form, the world will be free of hatred and would be overflowing with love. When love takes over, it brings Abundance of Happiness.

Happiness looks different for everyone. For you, maybe it's being at peace with who you are. Or having a secure network of friends who accept you unconditionally. Or the freedom to pursue your deepest dreams.

Regardless of your version of true happiness, living a happier, more satisfying life is within reach.

Chapter One

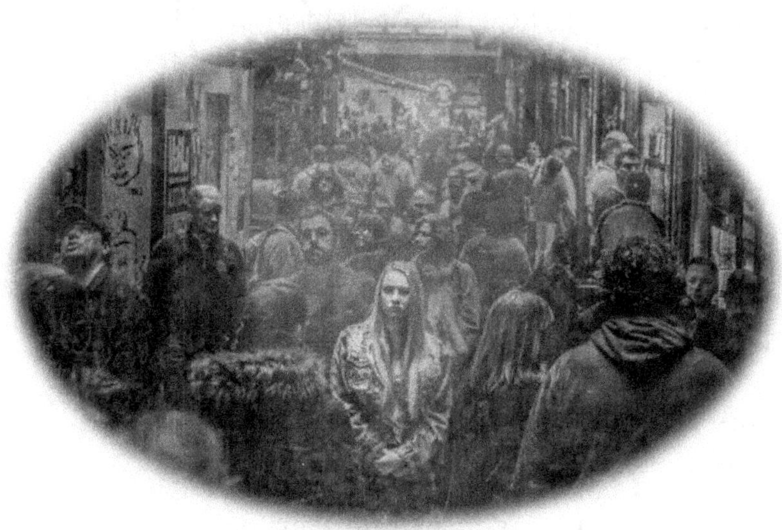

Why Are We Unhappy?

With the advance of modern technology, life has become easier, people have more money and comforts. Why then the majority of us are unhappy in some way or the other? I think the reason for our unhappiness is that we have become too materialistic. We are more focused on gathering material things. Unfortunately, the desire for this is never-ending. It is an endless pit.

The modern-day progress has made our lives easier and comfortable but not any happier. That's because we are not enhancing our level of consciousness which would lead to the understanding of the things which matter.

Some of the reasons for our unhappiness could be:

Comparison with Others

There is this story about a peacock and a crow.

Once, there was a crow who lived in a forest and was satisfied in life. But one day he saw a beautiful swan and thought to himself, "This swan is so white and beautiful, and I am so black and hence unpleasant to the eye. This swan must be the happiest bird in the world."

He expressed his thoughts to the swan. "Actually," the swan replied, "I was feeling that I was the happiest bird around until I saw a parrot, which has two colours. I now think the parrot is the happiest bird in creation." The crow then approached the parrot. The parrot explained, "I lived a very happy life until I saw a peacock. I have only two colours, but the peacock has multiple colours."

The crow then visited a peacock in the zoo and saw that hundreds of people had gathered to see him. After the people had left, the crow approached the peacock. "Dear peacock," the crow said, "you are so beautiful. Every day thousands of people come to see you. When people see me, they immediately shoo me away. I think you are the happiest bird on the planet."

The peacock replied, "I always thought that I was the most beautiful and happy bird on the planet. But because of my beauty, I am entrapped in this zoo. I have examined the zoo very carefully, and I have realized that the crow is the only bird not kept in a cage. So, for the past few days, I have been thinking that if I were a crow, I could happily roam everywhere."

Comparison with ourselves brings improvement, comparison with others bring discontent.

Comparing ourselves with others will make us unhappy. We might inadvertently be comparing the strength of another person with our weaknesses, which would be unfair to ourselves. If you focus on your strengths, you will multiply them. However, if we focus on our weakness, at the best we will become mediocre and at the worst, frustrated.

Each one of us has a different journey to success. We have circumstances, obstacles, and opportunities. Each one of us has our unique abilities.

The right approach is to get inspired by others and not compare with them.

Real happiness comes from satisfaction. If we have given our best to whatever we are doing, we will have a sense of satisfaction, which is the real source of happiness.

The sense of 'I'm not enough" "I'm not rich enough", "beautiful enough"," smart enough" etc. creates sadness within ourselves. Keep saying to yourself "I'm enough".

You are stuck in your comfort zone

A comfort zone is a beautiful place, but nothing grows there.

The following poem by an anonymous poet sums up the story of the life of a person stuck in a comfort zone until he thought of venturing out.

I used to have a comfort zone where I knew I wouldn't fail. The same four walls and busywork were really more like jail.

I longed so much to do the things I'd never done before, But stayed inside my comfort zone and paced the same old floor

I said it didn't matter that I wasn't doing much. I said I didn't care for things like commission checks and such.

I claimed to be so busy with the things inside my zone, But deep inside I longed for something special of my own.

Fit as a Fiddle Happy as a Lark

*I couldn't let my life go by just watching others win.
I held my breath; I stepped outside and let the change
begin.*

*I took a step and with new strength, I'd never felt before,
I kissed my comfort zone good-bye and closed and locked
the door*

*If you're in the comfort zone, afraid to venture out,
Remember that all winners were at one time filled with
doubt.*

**A step or two and words of praise can make your dreams
came true**

*Reach for your future with a smile;
Success is there for you!*

One of the most common reasons for the lack of happiness in people's lives is a lack of growth. At some point in time in our lives, we get stuck in our comfort zone. Most of us try to play safe all the time and call this 'being practical'.

We don't pull up our courage to do what we want to do or what we must do to progress. We don't put efforts to realise our dreams, or worse still, we don't dare to dream at all.

All our lives we live a mediocre life and regret when it is too late. Most common remorse of people on their death bed is that they wished they dared to live a life true to themselves and not the life others expected of them.

Sometimes we think that we are too young or too old for trying out something different. At other times we think that our circumstances are not right yet. There are times when we think too much about what if we fail. The lack of courage to come out of our comfort zone makes us unhappy about our lives.

Not being in the present moment

We are either brooding over our past or worrying about our future. This whole focus on past and future makes us unable to enjoy our present moment and that becomes the reason for our unhappiness.

This incident given below will tell us the difference in the attitude of a person annoyed at the past and anxious about the future and someone who lives in the present.

On a busy Monday morning, the young mom shouted out at her husband, "Honey, would you drop the kids off to school today? I've got a lot of chores to complete and errands to run."

Not too happy with the request the husband agreed in a grumbling tone. He yelled at the kids, "Hurry up, kids! I don't have all day."

So, the father and the kids jumped into the car and drove off. The busy father glancing at his watch fumed. *"My wife could have easily finished off her chores yesterday when it was a holiday. This last-minute task is going to make me late for work. My boss won't be too happy about it. What if he's already in a bad mood?"*

While he was complaining about the past and worrying about the future, his car approached a railway crossing. Just as he reached there, the safety gate closed down right in front of him. As expected, he banged his fist on the dashboard and groaned saying, *"Dammit! I'm going to be held up by a train and be delayed further."*

As the dad was fuming in the front seat, anxiously tapping his fingers on the steering wheel, reviewing, in his mind, how to make up some time … a sweet little voice of a child, calls out from the backseat: *"Daddy, Daddy, we're so lucky! We get to watch the train go by!"*

The point to remember is that we can't ever go back and undo the action of the past. Similarly, we cannot go to the future and make things happen now.

The only place where we can be is, in the present. Being in the present is very relaxing. Just as the child in the present was happy and relaxed as against his father who was stressed.

Be in the present with all your senses. Listen to the sounds, observe the colours and shapes of the things around. Feel the texture of the things you touch; taste the food you eat. Be aware of the smells.

"If you are depressed you are living in the past. If you are anxious you are living in the future. If you are at peace you are living in the present."

- Lao Tzu

Tying your happiness to something or someone

Most people think that happiness is possible only on the happening of certain events and not before. You must have heard statements like the ones below from others, and you might have found yourself thinking these thoughts: I'll be happy when I own a luxury car, a big house, or a perfect partner or when I have a big fat bank account. I'll be happy when I have the latest version of the iPhone. Diamonds will make me happy. A certain Job or a certain place will make me happy.

What's common in all the above statements?

In all such cases, we tie our happiness to the happening of some event or certain material possession. This makes our happiness conditional.

Setting a criterion for our happiness is like running after a mirage. Once you reach a certain point, you start to look for something more. And hence happiness keeps eluding us.

Does that mean we should not have goals or dreams? Of course not. On the contrary, it's wonderful to think big and go after big goals. There is nothing wrong with that. The problem is when we tie our happiness with the happening of those events, we put ourselves into a vicious circle because we set conditions for our happiness.

The best way is to get excited about and strive to achieve the goal, but at the same time, be joyful and enjoy the journey.

So, what should we do? I believe that our objective should be to attain the level of happiness which is unconditional.

"I am determined to be cheerful and happy in whatever situation I may find myself. For I have learned that the greater part of our misery or unhappiness is determined not by our circumstance but by our disposition."
-Martha Washington

Unconditional happiness is something that should be our ultimate goal because then you can control it on your own. You can be happy right here and now.

You don't need any big material possessions or other people or any other conditions to become happy. You can just become happier in the present moment.

Fit as a Fiddle Happy as a Lark

Being happy in no manner means not being sincere or serious about your goals; being happy increases your chances of achieving your goals.

Chapter Two

Rituals for Creating Happiness

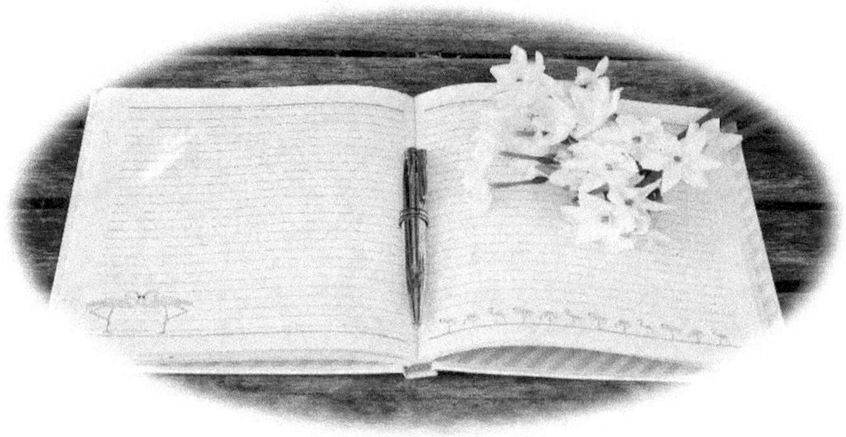

Establishing rituals is of paramount importance if you want to break the old habit patterns which make you unhappy and imbibe new habits which make you happy. If you've ever tried breaking a bad habit, you know all too well how ingrained it is. Well, good habits are deeply engrained, too. Why not work on making positive habits a part of your routine?

Let's take a look at some daily, monthly, and yearly habits to help kickstart your quest. Just remember that everyone's version of happiness is a little different, and so is their path to achieving it. If some of these habits create added stress or just don't fit into your lifestyle, ditch them. With a little time and practice, you'll figure out what does and doesn't work for you.

Project Happiness

"Smiling is the best way to face every problem, to crush every fear, and to hide every pain."

-Will Smith

Smile. Even if you are not happy, act as if you are. You tend to smile when you're happy however, it's actually a two-way street. We smile because we're happy, and smiling causes the brain to release dopamine, which makes us happier.

That doesn't mean you have to go around with a fake smile plastered on your face all the time. But the next time you find yourself feeling low, crack a smile, and see what happens. Or try starting each morning by smiling at yourself in the mirror.

Smile

we crack a smile—a genuine eye crinkle which is called a "Duchenne smile"—our cardiovascular system calms.

Laughing takes it one step further. Partly because it forces us to exhale. Simply exhaling lowers our heart rate and induces feelings of calm.

Smiling releases endorphins, which combat stress hormones. My **suggestion** is, "You should practice smiling right now, even if you feel foolish. You're cancelling some of the stress cortisol and you're increasing your happiness—a double bonus." So, enjoy the funny side.

Move your Body

Exercise isn't just for your body. Regular exercise can help to reduce stress, anxiety, and feelings of depression while boosting self-confidence, self-esteem, and happiness.

Even a small amount of regular physical activity can make a sea of difference in the long run. You don't have to train for a triathlon or scale a cliff — unless of course if that's what makes you happy. The trick is not to overexert. If you suddenly throw yourself into a strenuous routine, you'll probably just end up frustrated and sore.

Consider these exercise starters:

1. Take a walk around the block every night after dinner.

2. Sign up for a beginner's class in yoga or aerobics.

3. Start your day with 5 minutes of stretching.

Remind yourself of any fun activities you once enjoyed, but that has fallen by the wayside. Or activities you always wanted to try, such as golf, swimming, or dancing.

Reboot yourself with quality sleep

"There is only one thing people like that is good for them; a good night's sleep."
                                        -E. W. Howe

No matter how much modern society steers us toward less sleep, we know that adequate sleep is a vital trusted source to good health, brain function, and emotional well-being.

Most adults need about 7 or 8 hours of sleep every night. If you find yourself fighting the urge to nap during the day or just generally feel like you're in a fog, your body may be telling you it needs more rest.

Fit as a Fiddle Happy as a Lark

Here are a few tips to help you build a better sleep routine:

1. Write down how many hours of sleep you get each night and how rested you feel. After a week, you should have a better idea of how you're doing.

2. As the saying goes "Early to bed and early to rise makes a person healthy, wealthy and wise", hence, go to bed and wake up at the same time every day, including weekends.

3. Reserve the hour before bed as quiet time. Take a bath, read a book, listen to some relaxing music or do something to unwind yourself.

4. Avoid heavy eating and drinking before bedtime.

5. Keep your bedroom dark, cool, and quiet.

6. Invest in a good mattress.

7. If you have to take a nap during the day, try to limit it to 20 minutes.

If you consistently have problems sleeping, consult your doctor.

Breathe deeply

You're tensed, your shoulders are tight, and you feel as though you just might collapse. We all know that feeling. Instinct may tell you to take a long, deep breath to calm yourself down. Turns out, that instinct is a good one.

According to Harvard Health, deep breathing exercises can help reduce stress.

The next time you feel stressed or are at your wit's end, work through these steps:

1. Close your eyes. Try to envision a happy memory or a beautiful place.
2. Take a slow, deep breath.
3. Slowly breathe out through your mouth.
4. Repeat this process several times, until you start to feel calm.

If you're having a hard time taking slow, deliberate breaths, try counting to 5 in your head with each inhales and exhales.

Acknowledge the unhappy moments

A positive attitude is generally a good thing, but bad things happen to everyone. It's just part of life. If you get some bad news, make a mistake, or just feel like you are stuck, don't try to pretend you're happy.

Acknowledge the feeling of unhappiness, letting yourself experience it for a moment. Then, shift your focus toward what made you feel this way and what it might take to recover. Would a deep breathing exercise help? A long walk outside? Talking it over with someone? Let the moment pass and take care of yourself. Remember, no one's happy all the time.

Keep a journal

"Journaling is like whispering to one's self and listening at the same time."

-Mina Murray

A journal is a good way to organize your thoughts, analyse your feelings, and make plans. And you don't have to be a literary genius or write volumes to benefit. It can be as simple as jotting down a few thoughts before you go to bed. If putting certain things in writing makes you nervous, you can always shred it when you've finished. It's the process that counts.

Declutter

"Clutter is the physical manifestation of unmade decisions fuelled by procrastination."

—Christina Scalise

Decluttering sounds like a big project, but setting aside just 20 minutes a week can have a big impact. Decluttering doesn't happen overnight. It's a process—and often, one that requires equal parts motivation and inspiration.

What can you do in 20 minutes? Lots. Here are some tips.

1. Set a timer on your phone and take 15 minutes to tidy up a specific area of one room — say, your closet or that out-of-control junk drawer. Put everything in its place and toss or give away any extra clutter that's not serving you anymore.
2. Keep a designated box for giveaways to make things a little easier (and avoid creating more clutter).
3. Use the remaining 5 minutes to do a quick walk through your living space, putting away whatever stray items end up in your path.

You can do this trick once a week, once a day, or anytime you feel like your space is getting out of control.

See Friends

Socialize- Join some club, connect with your old friends, make new friends. Humans are social beings, and having close friends can make us happier. Who do you miss? Reach out to them. Make a date to get together or simply have a long phone chat. In adulthood, it can feel next to impossible to make new friends. But it's not about how many friends you have. It's about having meaningful relationships — even if it's just with one or two people.

Try getting involved in a local volunteer group or taking a class. Both can help to connect you with like-minded people in your area. And chances are, they're looking for friends, too. Companionship doesn't have to be limited to other humans. Pets can offer similar benefits. Love animals but can't have a pet? Consider volunteering at a local animal shelter to make some new friends — both human and animal.

However, you must choose your friends carefully. You are the average of the five friends you hang out with. Choosing your friends wisely is one of the most important factors related to happiness. Do you have some friends who are energy vampires? **Energy vampires are those who drain your energy** when you're around them. Perhaps they're frequently complaining and reminding you of negative events? **Try to stay away** from such toxic people, and **mingling** with optimistic people, who make you feel **positive and energized**. Purchasing material items like televisions, clothes, jewellery, and cars won't make you happier. All they do is give momentary happiness. **Humans beings are social animals. We derive happiness and satisfaction from social connections.** Hence, I suggest that we invest time and money in people who contribute to our growth. Socialise, spend some quality time with family, friends, colleagues. Go for outings, concerts, yoga retreat, a holiday to some exotic destination, etc.

Plan your week

"If you fail to plan, you are planning to fail!"

- Benjamin Franklin

Feel like you're flailing about? Sit down at the end of every week and make a basic list for the following week. Even if you don't stick to the plan, blocking out time where you can do laundry, go grocery shopping, or tackle projects at work can help to quiet your mind.

You can get a fancy planner, but even a sticky note on your computer or piece of scrap paper in your pocket can do the job.

Unplug

"Being connected to everything has disconnected us from ourselves and the preciousness of this present moment."

— L.M. Browning

Ditch your phone. Turn off all the electronics and put those earbuds away for at least one hour once a week. They'll still be there for you later. If you still want them, that is.

If you haven't unplugged in a while, you might be surprised at the difference it makes. Let your mind wander free for a change. Read. Meditate. Take a walk and pay attention to your surroundings. Be sociable. Or be alone. Just be.

Sounds too daunting? Try doing a shorter amount of time several times a week.

Find a self-care ritual

"Love yourself first, and everything else falls in line. You really have to love yourself to get anything done in this world."

- Lucille Ball

It's easy to neglect self-care in a fast-paced world. However, since your body carries your thoughts, passions, and spirit through this world, doesn't it deserve a little love?

Maybe it's unwinding your workweek with a long, hot bath. Or adopting a skincare routine that makes you feel indulgent. Or simply setting aside a night to put on your softest jammies and watch a movie from start to finish. A relaxing massage once a week can do wonders for your body and mind.

Whatever it is, make time for it. Put it in your planner if you must, but do it.

Treat Yourself to a day out

"You have to treat yourself every once in a while, get to the fun stuff!"

-Heidi Klum

No one to go out with? Well, what rule says you can't go out alone? Go to your favourite restaurant, watch a movie, or go on that trip you've always dreamed of. Even if you're a social butterfly, spending some deliberate time alone can help you reconnect with the activities that truly make you happy.

Take time to reflect

"Life can only be understood backward, but it must be lived forward."

-Soren Kierkegaard

The start of a new year is a good time to stop and take inventory of your life. Set aside some time to catch up with yourself the way you would with an old friend and introspect on the following:

1. How are you doing?

2. What have you been up to?

3. Are you happier than you were a year ago?

Please avoid the pitfalls of judging yourself too harshly for your answers. You've made it to another year, and that itself is plenty.

If you find that your mood hasn't improved much over the last year, consider hiring a coach or making an appointment with a counsellor or talking to a therapist. You might be dealing with depression or even an underlying physical condition that's impacting your mood. To rule that out it would be wise to consult a doctor.

Re-evaluate your goals

"You have to keep recycling yourself."
-Chuck Palahniuk

People change, so think about where you're heading and consider if that's still where you want to go. There's no shame in changing your game.

Let go of any goals that no longer serve you, even if they sound nice on paper.

Fit as a Fiddle Happy as a Lark

Take care of your body

 It's been said that a healthy mind resides in a healthy body. Your physical and mental health are closely intertwined. You will find plenty of tips for your physical health in the first section of this book.

Chapter Three

Making Space for Happiness

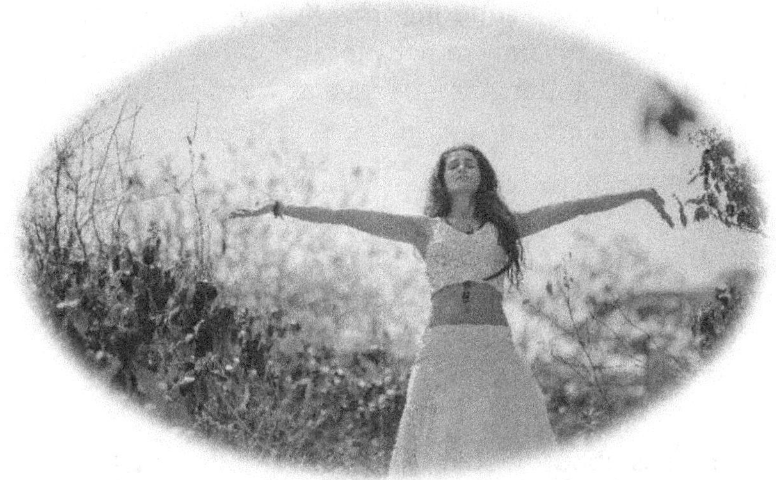

To make space for happiness we need to get rid of some of the rubbish we have collected in our life. Following are some of the ways to cleanse your heart and refurbish it.

Forgiveness

When another person hurts us, it can overturn our lives. Sometimes the hurt is very deep, especially when a spouse or a parent betrays our trust, or when we are victims of a crime, or when we've been harshly bullied. Anyone who has suffered a grievous hurt knows that when our inner world is badly disrupted, it's difficult to concentrate on anything other than our turmoil or pain. When we hold on to hurt, we are emotionally crippled, and our relationships suffer. This leads to profound unhappiness. We have two choices, one to self- sabotage with self-pity and suffering or forgive and let go. Forgiveness is the only remedy for this. When life hits us hard, there is nothing as effective as forgiveness for healing deep wounds. I am saying this from my own experience.

Agreed, the suffering may have had a deep impact on your life, your peace of mind, however, 'letting go' of these feelings will help you move on with life with a renewed vigour and hope.

 Forgiveness is about goodness, about extending mercy to those who've harmed us, even if they don't deserve it. It is not about finding excuses for the offending person's behaviour or pretending it didn't happen. Nor is there a quick formula you can follow. Forgiveness is a process which involves efforts. However, it's worth it. Working on forgiveness can help us increase our self-esteem and give us a sense of inner strength and safety. It can reverse the lies that we often tell ourselves when someone has hurt us deeply—lies like, "*I am defeated*" or "*I'm not worthy.*" Forgiveness can heal us and allow us to move on in life with meaning and purpose. Forgiveness matters, and we will be its primary beneficiary.

It's important to figure out who has hurt you and how. This may seem obvious, but not every action that causes you suffering is unjust. For example, you don't need to forgive your child or your spouse for being imperfect, even if their imperfections are inconvenient for you.

Forgiveness is always hard when we are dealing with deep injustices from others. I have known people who refuse to use the word forgiveness because it just makes them so angry. That's OK—we all have our timelines for when we can be merciful. But if you want to forgive and are finding it hard you can try Metta meditation.

First remember that if you are struggling with forgiveness, that doesn't mean you're a failure at forgiveness. Forgiveness is a process that takes time, patience, and determination. Try not to be harsh on yourself, but be gentle and foster a sense of quiet within, an inner acceptance of yourself. Try to respond to yourself as you would to someone whom you love deeply.

Surround yourself with good and wise people who support you and who have the patience to allow you time to heal in your way. Also, practice humility—not in the sense of putting yourself down, but in realizing that we are all capable of imperfection and suffering.

Try to develop courage and patience in yourself to help you in the journey. Also, if you practice bearing small slights against you without lashing out, you give a gift to everyone—not only to the other person but to everyone whom that person may harm in the future because of your anger. You can help end the cycle of inflicting pain on others.

If you are still finding it hard to forgive, you can choose to practice with someone easier to forgive—maybe someone who hurt you in a small way, rather than deeply. Alternatively, it can be better to focus on forgiving the person who is at the root of your pain—maybe an abusive parent or a spouse who betrayed you. If these hurts impact other parts of your life and other relationships, it may be necessary to start there.

Forgive yourself. Most of us tend to be harder on ourselves than we are on others and we struggle to love ourselves. If you are not feeling lovable because of some things you have done, you may need to work on self-forgiveness and offer to yourself what you offer to others who have hurt you: a sense of inherent worth, despite your actions.

In self-forgiveness, you honour yourself as a person, even if you are imperfect. If you've seriously broken your standards, there is a danger of sliding into self-loathing. When this happens, you may not take good care of yourself—you might overeat or oversleep or start smoking or engage in other forms of "self-punishment." You need to recognize this and move toward self-compassion. Soften your heart toward yourself.

After you have been able to self-forgive, you will also need to engage in seeking forgiveness from others whom you've harmed and right the wrongs as best as you can. It's important to be prepared for the possibility that the other person may not be ready to forgive you and to practice patience and humility. But, a sincere apology, free of conditions and expectations, will go a long way toward your receiving forgiveness in the end.

Metta Meditation

Develop Metta (Loving Kindness)

Metta is the practice of cultivating *universal* love, friendliness, or lovingkindness. Metta is benevolence toward all beings, without discrimination or selfish attachment. Metta can be compared to the *unconditional love* that a mother would have for her children. This love does not discriminate between benevolent people and malicious people. It is a love in which "I" and "you" disappear, and where there is no possessor and nothing to possess. By practising Metta, one can overcome anger, ill will, hatred and aversion. It is an excellent meditation for forgiveness and letting go of grudges.

The practice progresses in five stages. As we use Metta during meditation, we cultivate Metta for:
1. Ourselves
2. A good friend
3. A neutral person — someone we don't have any strong feelings for

4. A difficult person — someone we have conflicts with or feelings of ill will towards
5. All sentient beings

In your practice, you can access Metta through meditation and identifying someone at each of the stages. Learning to accept all for how they are will give you the freedom to love and forgive.

Metta Meditation Script

1. Find a comfortable position in which to sit for this period. As you allow your eyes to gently close, tune into the body and make any minor adjustments. It can be helpful to remember our intentions of both ease and awareness. Sit in a way that feels comfortable but alert.

2. We'll start with a few minutes of concentration practice, just to help our minds settle and arrive in our present time experience.

3. As you allow the body to resume to natural breathing, see where in the body you can feel the breath. It may be in the stomach or abdomen, where you can feel the rising and falling as we breathe. It might be in the chest, where you may notice the expansion and contraction as the body inhales and exhales. Perhaps it's at the nostrils, where you can feel a slight tickle as the air comes in, and the subtle warmth as the body exhales. You can pick one spot to stick with for this meditation practice.

4. As you feel the body breathing, try to stay with the breath all the way through. Stick with it from the beginning of the inhale through the end of the exhale. (Allow for some silence here for as long as you see fit)

5. You may have noticed the mind wandering. When the mind wanders, it offers us an opportunity to cultivate mindfulness and concentration. Each time we notice the mind wandering, we're strengthening our ability to recognize our experience. Each time we bring the mind back to the breath, we're strengthening our ability to focus on an object. Treat it as an opportunity rather than a problem, and return to the breath. (Allow for some silence here for as long as you see fit)

6. You can begin the practice by bringing to mind yourself as you sit here right now. Try to connect with your own deepest intentions for happiness, ease, and safety. You don't need to dive into stories of what will make you happy but connect with that natural desire you have. You can cultivate this intention to open the heart to your wellbeing by silently offering yourself some phrases of Metta. In your head, slowly offer yourself the phrases: "May I be happy." "May I be healthy." "May I be safe." "May I be at ease." You

can offer these phrases silently in your head, saying them slowly enough so that you can connect with their meaning and the intention behind them. (Allow for some silence here for as long as you see fit)

7. You can now bring to mind a good friend. This may be a loved one, a friend, a teacher or mentor, or maybe a pet. You can connect with your natural desire to see this person happy and at ease. Just like you, this person wants to be happy, to feel safe, and to be healthy. To cultivate this intention of kindness, you can offer this person a few phrases of Metta: "May you be happy." "May you be healthy." "May you be safe." "May you be at ease." (Allow for some silence here for as long as you see fit)

8. You can let this person go from your mind and bring to mind a neutral person. This is someone you see, maybe regularly, but don't know very well. It may be somebody who works somewhere you go a lot, a co-worker, or maybe a neighbour. Although you don't know this person well, you can recognize that this person wants to be happy as well. You don't need to know what their happiness looks like necessarily. Again, offer this person the phrases of loving-kindness, connecting to care about their wellbeing. "May you be happy." "May you be healthy." "May you be

safe." "May you be at ease." (Allow for some silence here for as long as you see fit)

9. And as you let this neutral person go, you can bring to mind somebody who you find difficult. You may not want to pick the most difficult person in your life, instead choosing someone who is minorly difficult. Maybe it's someone you find yourself agitated with or annoyed by. Again, offer this person the phrases of loving-kindness, connecting to care about their wellbeing. "May you be happy." "May you be healthy." "May you be safe." "May you be at ease." (Allow for some silence here for as long as you see fit)

Let go of Grudges

This is often easier said than done. But you don't have to do it for the other person. Sometimes, offering forgiveness or dropping a grudge is about compassion towards self and not just for others.

Take some time and assess your relationships with others. Are you harbouring any resentment or ill-will toward someone? If so, consider reaching out to them to bury the hatchet. This doesn't have to be a reconciliation. You may just need to end the relationship and move on.

If reaching out isn't an option, try getting your feelings out in a letter. You don't even have to send it to them.

Just getting your feelings out of your mind and into the world can be freeing.

Travel Light

Drop your emotional baggage. The burden of our heavy past should be abandoned. Life is a journey and we can't carry everything with us. Only carry the useful stuff.

You've probably heard of the fear of missing out but what about the fear of letting go?

My father was volatile and aggressive. Criticism was his preferred method of communication. As a child and teenager, I learned to keep my thoughts and feelings locked away. Without realizing it, I carried this habit into adulthood, avoiding any talk about my feelings or turning them into a joke. When a friend finally called me on it, the shock of self-recognition quickly turned to resistance. *'This is who I am'*, I thought. *'Why should I change?'*

I trod on, working as hard as ever to keep my fortress intact. It wasn't making me happy yet I wasn't ready to change. As I struggled with my desire to cling to hurtful memories and self-defeating behaviours, it dawned on me that I was afraid to let go because defensiveness was part of my identity.

The problem wasn't that I had baggage—everyone has baggage. The problem was that, it had come to define me. I didn't know who I would be without it. At that point, it hit me: I had to dig deep, discover the person I wanted to be, and then *act* on it.

After I identified that I was holding on to the past because it seemed too important to jettison, I discovered that letting go is harder than it sounds. Relaxing a long-held belief isn't a one-day, one-week, or even a one-year process. However, it *is* possible.

This is the five-step process you can follow:
1. Write an honest list of the thoughts, beliefs, and behaviours that weigh you down. Grab a pen and notebook, find a quiet space, and spend thirty to forty minutes thinking and writing. It is important, to be honest, and write down whatever comes to mind. Don't judge what comes up, just take note.

2. Reflect on each item and identify the source of the thought. Travel back in time and see where you picked up these items of baggage. Do you fear intimacy because a partner cheated on you? Do you dread the holidays because your parents fought all the time? Acknowledge the painful memories but don't wallow in them. Write them down and move on to the next step.

3. Find at least one positive thing in each hurtful experience. Look for the silver lining in your cloud. For example, my father's criticism made me aware of the power of words and taught me the importance of speaking with kindness. Looking for the good in the past helps you reclaim your

power. You are no longer a victim. *You* decide what you take from that experience.

4. Create affirmations to foster change and counteract negative thoughts. Take the positives from step three and turn them into affirmations or statements of intent, i.e.: "I will speak with love" or "I will treat people with kindness." This emphasizes positive future behaviour and frees you from the past. Make the affirmations tangible: put a reminder on your phone, write them on post-its, or put a list on the fridge.

5. Practice patience and mindfulness. It takes time to change habits, especially when they are rooted in deep hurts or fears. Check-in with yourself regularly using journaling or meditation. If you find yourself shouldering old baggage, be sure to acknowledge it, then gently release it and focus on your affirmations. Replacing negative thoughts with positive actions will help you let go for good.

There are infinite possibilities for each of us, baggage notwithstanding. Everyone has pain. It's part of what makes us who we are. What defines us, however, is how we handle it.

One of my favourite artists, Bruce Springsteen, has some wise words on the subject: *"You can find your identity in the damage that's been done to you. You find your identity in your wounds, in your scars, in the places where you've been beaten up and you turn them into a medal.*

We all wear the things we've survived with some honour, but the real honour is in also transcending them."

By taking the time to identify and understand our baggage and making a conscious decision to let go, we free ourselves to experience life in a richer, deeper, more meaningful way.

Gratitude

Simply being grateful can give your mood a big boost, among other benefits. For example, a recent two-part study done in the psychology department of the Hope College in the USA in 2016, found that practising gratitude can have a significant impact on feelings of hope and happiness.

Start each day by acknowledging one thing you're grateful for. You can do this while you're brushing your teeth or just waiting for that snoozed alarm to go off again.

As you go about your day, try to keep an eye out for pleasant things in your life. They can be big things, such as knowing that someone loves you or getting a well-deserved promotion. They can also be little things, such as a co-worker who offered you a cup of coffee or the neighbour who waved to you. Maybe even just the warmth of the sun on your skin.

With a little practice, you may even become more aware of all the positive things around you.

Why do we lack Gratitude?

One of the biggest reasons for feeling unhappy or sad is that we don't count our blessings when we wake up every day. Rather, we focus on the things we lack and believe that our happiness is solely dependent on achieving the next big thing.

We have so many examples in life to prove that happiness from every next physical thing in only short-lived. The moment we get what we are looking for, we again start looking at something bigger than that

If you are consistently focussing on the lack in your life, it will create a never fulfilling mental loop.

"What you focus on grows, what you think about expands and what you dwell upon determines your reality"

-Robin Sharma

You think the glass is half empty. You don't feel grateful that even this half glass can quench your thirst.

One shouldn't make his or her happiness solely dependent on the achievement of the materialistic goals. If you have a house to stay, a vehicle to drive, a reasonable job or a vocation to lead a nice life with your family, you are already better off than a substantial population.

Your gratitude has a positive impact on your future too. Because:

"What you appreciate, appreciates"

-Lynee Twist

What can we appreciate in our day to day life?

1. When you put toothpaste on your toothbrush, think of 1 thing that makes you feel grateful.

2. When you wake up in the morning, glance at a photo that makes you feel happy.

3. think of one good thing from your day at night.

Expressing thanks may be one of the simplest ways to feel better. Gratitude unshackles us from toxic emotions.

In positive psychology research, gratitude is strongly and consistently associated with greater happiness. Gratitude helps people feel more positive emotions, relish good experiences, improve their health, deal with adversity, and build strong relationships.

People feel and express gratitude in multiple ways. They can apply it to the past by retrieving positive memories and being thankful for elements of childhood or past blessings. They can apply it to the present by not taking good fortune for granted as it comes. And they can apply it to the future by maintaining a hopeful and optimistic attitude. Regardless of the inherent or current level of someone's gratitude, it's a quality that individuals can successfully cultivate further.

Ways to cultivate gratitude

Gratitude is a way for people to appreciate what they have instead of always reaching for something new in the hopes it will make them happier, or thinking they can't feel satisfied until every physical and material need is met. Gratitude helps people refocus on what they have instead of what they lack. And, although it may feel contrived at first, this mental state grows stronger with use and practice.

Here are some ways in which you can make cultivation of gratitude a daily habit.

Write a thank-you note. You can make yourself happier and nurture your relationship with another person by writing a thank-you letter expressing your enjoyment and appreciation of that person's impact on your life. Send it, or better yet, deliver and read it in person if possible. Make a habit of sending at least one gratitude letter a month. Once in a while, write one to yourself.

Thank someone mentally. No time to write? It may help just to think about someone who has done something nice for you and mentally thank the individual.

Keep a gratitude journal. Make it a habit to write down or share with a loved one, thoughts about the gifts you've received each day.

Count your blessings. Pick a time every week to sit down and write about your blessings — reflecting on what went right or what you are grateful for. Sometimes it helps to pick a number — such as three to five things — that you will identify each week. As you write, be specific and think about the sensations you felt when something good happened to you.

Pray. Religious people can use prayer to cultivate gratitude.

Hawaiian Forgiveness Mantra: Ho'oponopono

Another beautiful technique useful in developing a forgiving heart is 'Ho'oponopono', a powerful Hawaiian forgiveness mantra.

What is Ho'oponopono? And how does it help? Ho'oponopono is an ancient Hawaiian practise still in use today and is well-known for the miracle it does in clearing negativity from one's mind and thought. It is believed to be designed to wipe out all the negativity in our thoughts and those blocks that are keeping us miserable.

Dr Joe Vitale is a renowned Ho'oponopono practitioner, He says that there are a large number of us who don't have the luxury of enjoying peace, harmony or joy forever in our lives. It is believed that external negativity plays a role and we are saddled right from our birth. This Hawaiian technique Ho'oponopono has been specifically designed to remove all the stress and negativity from our minds and let us enjoy eternal happiness. It is a simple technique where you ask for forgiveness and purify yourself.

There are four phases or steps that we can follow and the magical healing starts from within. The four steps involved in this practice make you realize the fact that you are responsible for everything that happens to you and that is in your mind. Once you realize this fact it becomes easy for you to start practising the steps.

1. The first step asks you to say sorry for everything that has happened or any wrong things that you have witnessed. It makes easy for you to move ahead in your life once you know the fact and has the courage to say sorry for anything that was wrong, you will feel better.

2. Once you are able to say sorry the second step requires you to ask for forgiveness. You will be seeking forgiveness for everything you felt sorry for in the first step. While doing so you are asking to forgive everything from you and your past memories that may have been involved in the wrongdoing. These may sound weird for many of us but once you mean what you say the process is magical.

3. The third step that you must go through is showing your gratitude for everything that has happened to your life. This way you will learn to appreciate everything that is big or small in your life. You might get an unexpected response for this thank you but you need not worry about the result or response. In right time the correct result will appear in front of you. This step will help you to have patience as well.

4. The last step that you need to follow is to show your love and say I love you to everything that is yours. This way you will learn to love everything related to you.

What's Ho'oponopono theory of magic that will help you can be elaborated further with the effect that each step has on you. It makes you stronger and gives you the courage to face the truth and tell the truth. You will feel better when you know that your request for the forgiveness has been granted and people are going to trust you again. There is no human being on the planet who does not commit sins either knowingly or unknowingly. The ones who dare to see their mistake, and come forward to seek forgiveness are the successful ones. Live your life with no grudges and you will be the happiest person.

There are four sentences to this technique or meditation or prayer whatever you may like to call it. These sentences are so simple that we find it hard to believe in the miracles that they can achieve. Repentance, Forgiveness, Gratitude and Love are the only forces at work here and these forces have amazing power.

The best part of chanting this mantra is that you can do it by yourself. You don't need anyone else to be with you nor do you need anyone to hear you. You can chant the words in your head. The power is in our feeling it and in our willingness to forgive and love.

Chant the following either aloud or in your mind. Chant it for as long as you want to or you can, use a string of 108 beads and chant it while passing the beads through your fingers in the ancient Indian style.

These rather simple but, tremendously powerful words are:

I'M SORRY - PLEASE FORGIVE ME - THANK YOU - I LOVE YOU

The practice makes you love everything that belongs to you. This is important in the sense that people do not tend to care about the things and people that are making their life beautiful. You must show your appreciation for what you have and this will make the bonding stronger. Life is not about yourself but everyone and everything that are connected to you as well. It is necessary you take life as one beautiful chance given to you and handle it with care.

It helps you forget all the bad memories associated with you as you move forward with the forgiveness achieved from your action and prayers. Once you are a regular practitioner of this process you know that life is more about having faith and courage to accept and face the truth. You will never feel the pressure of hiding the bad side of you, rather you will learn to come forward and express what you want to go away from your life. This way you will be living stress-free life with no regrets.

Chapter Four

Happiness is a Way of Life

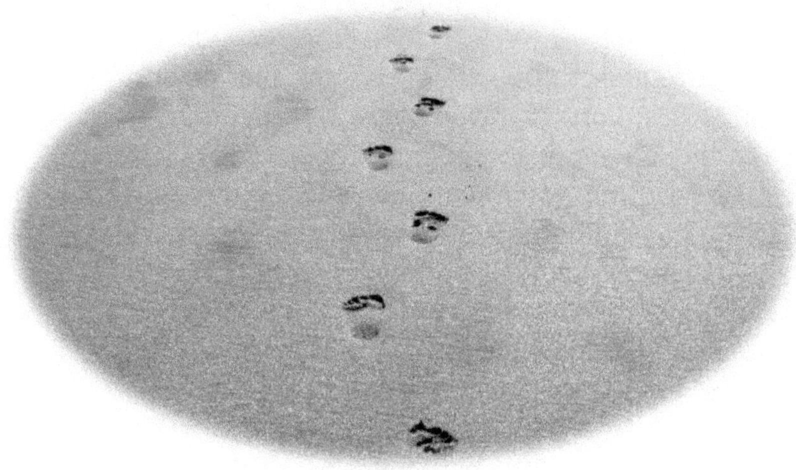

There are some qualities which you will have to purposefully cultivate and some things you will have to start doing if you wish to make happiness part of your personality.

I have listed some of them below:

Unwavering Faith

The dictionary meaning of Faith is *"a firm belief in something for which there is no proof"* or *"something that is believed especially with strong conviction."*

The world's top-most strategic coach, Tony Robbins, defines it as **"*certainty of outcome*"** in your mind when you are working towards your goals. He states that our success in any venture that we get into, entirely depends on the level of certainty of outcome in our minds, because only our thinking about the certainty of the outcome will trigger us to produce the quality of actions needed to get the results.

"*Faith is taking the first step, even if you don't see the whole staircase.*"

–*Martin Luther King, Jr.*

In addition to a strong belief in our abilities and a growth mindset, we need to develop a deeper sense of complete faith in the goodness of whatever happens in our life. Of course, it doesn't mean that when you have faith or believe strongly in the certainty of the outcome that you expect, you'll always achieve what you desire.

Many uncontrollable factors play a significant role, so despite your best efforts, sometimes you may not get the desired results.

But failures won't steal your happiness because you are already equipped with a growth mindset. Failure gives you the required experience and prompts you to develop the skill set necessary to handle the situation better.

Having faith means that, even if things don't go the way you desired, you believe in the bigger scheme of things. You believe in the unfolding of life towards a greater good for you. When you have faith, you strongly believe that things don't happen to you; they happen for you.

"Remember that sometimes, not getting what you want is a wonderful stroke of luck."

-Dalai Lama

You know that you can't control your genes or circumstances, but you can control your actions. You also realize that as you don't have full control over everything, so you are mindful that your happiness shouldn't solely depend on the outcome. Your happiness comes from taking action and getting immersed in the activities rather than overthinking about the past or future.

When you take consistent and massive action, you invite flow in your work, and your happiness is created by your immersion into the activities. So instead of waiting for some outcome to happen, to make you happier, you immediately experience happiness in the work you do. I'd say it's a win-win proposition. Because if you are joyful and get into the flow of whatever you do, there are great chances that the quality of your work will be multiple times better than when you are working under stress.

Finally, the objective of life is to strive for our goals, because growth is the need of our spirit, but at the same time, we need to ensure that we don't tie our momentary happiness to the achievement of those goals.

Do What You Love

Don't say, "I'll do what I love after I retire." Instead, plan on spending some time now, doing things you love. Even if it's a simple hobby. Decide when you can devote a little time regularly. If you don't like the work you're doing now, maybe you should consider a change of career.

When you find an activity that you enjoy, one that challenges you, and increases your skill, you'll find yourself fully engaged in it. You'll be in a flow state. This means you'll be concentrating on the present and may even lose your sense of time. This feels good and contributes to your well-being and happiness.

5.

Reframe Obstacles

No one gets through life without encountering obstacles. So, each time an obstacle pops up, try to reframe it as a challenge that you can handle. If you need support, think of a time when you surmounted your fear and successfully took action. Be a problem solver. You may ask yourself, 'How can I fix this?' Questioning opens the creative parts of your brain and you may come up with more than one solution. If life gives you a lemon, make lemonade.

Random Acts of Kindness

Practising acts of kindness gives people a happiness boost. Besides, the recipient becomes happier and this even extends to people who merely observe the act.

These acts could be anything from giving a smile, helping someone cross the road to gifting something handmade to a friend or loved one. It could also be assisting a family member with household chores. So please do more acts of kindness to make the world a happier place.

People perform acts of kindness both to do good and to feel good. Research finds that being kind makes us happy, helps to lower our blood pressure, and encourages stronger social connections. Now, a new study suggests that we can access some of these benefits simply by recalling acts of kindness we did in the past—making kindness a gift that keeps on giving.

Give a compliment. That's a beautiful act of kindness which does not cost you anything. Giving a sincere compliment is a quick, easy way to brighten someone's day while giving your own happiness a boost. Catch the person's eye and say it with a smile so they know you mean it. You might be surprised by how good it makes you feel. If you want to offer someone a compliment on their physical appearance, make sure to do it respectfully.

Practice 'Mudita'

'Mudita' means Sympathetic Joy. It is an important component of the Buddha's teachings. Mudita is taking sympathetic or altruistic joy in observance of the happiness of others. Mudita is the ability to take active delight in others' good fortune or good deeds as a way to develop and maintain calmness of mind. People also identify Mudita with empathy. The antithesis of Mudita is jealousy and envy which makes you unhappy.

By being happy when good things happen to others, your opportunities for delight are greatly increased. Practice Mudita when you observe the success and happiness in others.

Look your best

Dress well, be well-groomed, take frequent showers. Happy clothes include well-cut, figure-enhancing items made from bright and beautiful fabrics. Wear fancy jewellery, good quality makeup, splash on your favourite perfume. Men, do have a good haircut. Shave your beard or trim it. Have a manicure and a pedicure.

Recreation

Take up a hobby When it comes to improving your mental health, there are few better remedies than picking up a healthy hobby. Hobbies can get your mind active, and get you social—but the real benefit to most people is the boost to overall mental wellness. No matter what sort of mental issue you're struggling with, there's a good chance that throwing yourself into a hobby will have a positive effect on you. Listen to music, sing loudly even if it is in your bathroom, dance even if you are alone.

Our daily lives are filled with stress—from our jobs, our kids, school, bills, and relationship conflict to a seemingly endless list of other minor stressors. Hobbies play an important role in mitigating some of this unavoidable stress, as they provide us with an outlet for creativity, distraction, and something to look forward to.

Hobbies bring a sense of fun and freedom to life that can help to minimize the impact of chronic stress. Those who feel overwhelmed at a job, for example, can benefit from hobbies because they provide an outlet for stress and something to look forward to after a hard day or week at a stressful job.

Having a hobby to focus on forces us to take a break from stressful activities. Without a reason to take a break, we may unwittingly overwork ourselves to the point of exhaustion. Studies have shown that some of the best hobbies for reducing stress include knitting, gardening, reading, quilting, painting singing dancing and the list goes on.

Join a laughter yoga club

Laughter Yoga Clubs are social clubs that are free for all, anywhere in the world. Laughter Yoga is like an aerobic exercise (cardio workout) which brings more oxygen to the body and brain which makes one feel healthier and more energetic. Laughter Yoga strengthens the immune system.

 In India, most Laughter Clubs function on a daily basis and the members meet at public parks where people go for a morning walk. If you want to start a Laughter Club, find a place in your locality where people can assemble early morning while going for a walk. The concept of Laughter Clubs is slightly different in the West where club members like to meet for 1-2 hours every weekend or fortnightly. They laugh together for 30 minutes along with breathing and stretching exercises, followed by Laughter Meditation for 30 mins.

Back to Nature

We all know how good being in nature can make us feel. We have known it for centuries. The sounds of the forest, the scent of the trees, the sunlight playing through the leaves, the fresh, clean air — these things give us a sense of comfort. They ease our stress and worry, help us to relax and to think more clearly. Being in nature can restore our mood, give us back our energy and vitality, refresh and rejuvenate us.
Sometimes when I'm in the shower I imagine I'm washing away all my stress, negative feelings, sadness, remorse and anger. When I'm in the bathtub I imagine I'm soaking up love, appreciation warmth kindness care etc. When I bask in the sun, I imagine the sun is pouring joy, health prosperity etc on me. When I walk barefoot on the

ground, I imagine drawing strength, stability and energy from the earth.

Nature therapy sometimes referred to as ecotherapy, describes a broad group of techniques or treatments intending to improve an individual's mental or physical health, specifically with an individual's presence within nature or outdoor surroundings. One example of nature therapy is forest bathing or 'shinrin-yoku', a practice that combines a range of exercises and tasks in an outdoor environment.

If you're looking to reduce the stress of city life, escape to the forest and talk to the trees.

Concrete jungles create a lot of stress in our lives, which is why more and more people are turning to the gifts of nature for therapy — like tree-hugging, walking barefoot on the grass, mud or sand.

Hugging a tree increases levels of the hormone oxytocin. This hormone is responsible for feeling calm and emotional bonding. When hugging a tree, the hormones serotonin and dopamine make you feel happier. It is important to use this "free" space of a forest we were given by nature to holistically heal ourselves.

Life on earth is unimaginable without the Sun. Natural light is crucial for our health and well-being. The sunlight helps to regulate the natural rhythms of our body and not getting enough of it can impact our health in surprising ways. Exposure to sun rays also called sunbath therapy has been in use from ancient times due to its disease-fighting properties. Let's know what are the benefits of the sunbath.

Sunrays have several healing powers. They not only heal you physically but also emotionally. Remember the song by John Denver- *Sunshine on my shoulders makes me happy.* Breath Fresh air as often as you can. Try to drink natural spring water whenever you get a chance.

Face stress head-on

Life is full of stressors, and it's impossible to avoid all of them. For those stressors you can't avoid, remind yourself that everyone has stress — there's no reason to think it's all on you. And chances are, you're stronger than you think you are. Instead of letting yourself get overwhelmed, try to tackle the stressor head-on. This might mean initiating an uncomfortable conversation or putting in some extra work, but the sooner you tackle it, the sooner the pit in your stomach will start to shrink.

Look at Life as an Adventure

"Do not stop thinking of life as an adventure."
- Eleanor Roosevelt

Finally, if you think life as an adventure, you'll enjoy all the challenges coming in the way. Instead of avoiding, you'll move forward to seek those challenges.

Five Happiness Affirmations

'It's the repetition of affirmations that leads to belief. And once that belief becomes a deep conviction, things begin to happen.'

— Muhammad Ali

1. *"The Universe Supports Me."*
When you're feeling low or alone, it can be hard to feel as though anyone is on your side. This affirmation is a great reminder that you are never alone and that despite how things may seem, life is always on your side. The universe is continually orchestrating for things to work in your favour. You should keep having faith and your mind fixed firmly on what it is that you want most. Understand that these affirmations are going to become a reality for you.

2. *"I Am Enough."*
You are enough, exactly as you are right now. When you feel the pressures of life crashing down on you or you believe that happiness is only possible once you've achieved this, or look like that, it's time to bring yourself back to a place of self-love and know that you are always, already, enough.

3.   "My Heart Is Always Open and I Radiate Love."
Whether you're struggling with relationship problems, low self-esteem, work stresses or whatever it may be; you will always find that the best solution is rooted in love. So, use this as a reminder to always keep your heart open to giving and receiving love in all its forms.

4.   "I Have Everything I Need to Be Happy Right Now."
Gratitude is the most powerful tool there is for immediate, inner happiness. So, no matter what's going on around you, with this affirmation take a moment to reflect on everything you have to be grateful for and capture this feeling to see you through the rest of your day.

5.   "My Dreams Are Coming True Every Day."
Use this affirmation upon waking or the last thing at night, remind yourself of this until it becomes an integrated part of you.

A few more Affirmations for Happiness

1.   I choose to be happy and grateful today.

2.   Happiness flows through me constantly.

3.   My future is full of light and laughter.

4.   There are amazing things in my life; no matter how small they may seem, they are significant.

5.   I am at peace with my past.

Chapter Five

Happiness is a Journey Inwards

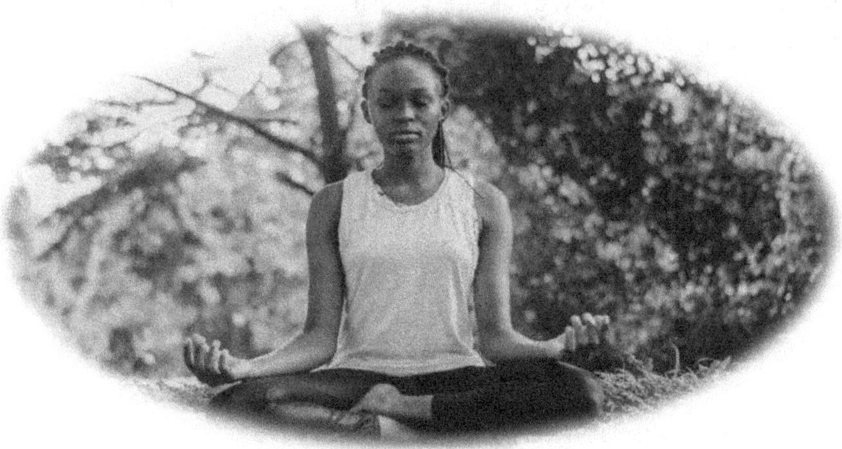

Meditation

You've probably heard that meditation can reduce stress, boost your immune system, and make you a happier, more focused person. But there are so many types of meditations, it can be hard to know which one will meet your needs.

What is meditation?

Meditation is an approach to training the mind, similar to the way that fitness is an approach to training the body.

Meditation is exploring. It's not a fixed destination. Your head doesn't become vacuumed free of thought immediately. It's a special place where each moment is momentous. When we meditate we venture into the workings of our minds: our sensations (air blowing on our skin or a harsh smell wafting into the room), our emotions (love this, hate that, crave this, loathe that) and thoughts (wouldn't it be weird to see an elephant playing the trumpet).

Many meditation techniques exist — so how do you learn how to meditate? It's extremely difficult for a beginner to sit for hours and think of nothing or have an "empty mind." However, there are plenty of meditation techniques for us to choose from.

The first step to starting a regular meditation practice is finding the style of meditation that's right for you. There are plenty of styles for you to choose from. You can try some of them and see which one suits you best. I have bellowed some of the techniques which I found helpful.

Where ever there are steps, script or instructions given for meditation in this book, you can either read out loud and record in your voice and play it. Or you could ask someone to read it for you. You can also go to my YouTube channel BodhiTreeLearnings and play the audio.

Anapana Sati Meditation

This one is my favourite. This is the meditation practice followed by the Buddha to attain Nirvana or

Enlightenment. This entails following the breath as we inhale and exhale. Breathing is something we do involuntarily as well as we can do it voluntarily that's why it is considered as the bridge between the conscious and the subconscious mind. If you do this with concentration and consistently, we can go to the alpha state. The alpha state of mind is when you reach a very relaxed state while awake. Another benefit of this meditation is that you can do it anytime and anywhere. 'Anapana Sati' makes you calm and aware.

Tratak Meditation

This meditation requires you to focus on a single point. staring at a candle flame, at the rising or the setting sun, a star, a dot, an idol etc. Since focusing the mind is challenging, a beginner might meditate for only a few minutes and then work up to longer durations. You simply refocus your awareness on the chosen object of attention each time you notice your mind wandering. Through this process, your ability to concentrate improves.

Mindfulness meditation

Mindfulness meditation asks us to suspend judgment and unleash our natural curiosity about the workings of the mind, approaching our experience with warmth and kindness, to ourselves and others.

Mindfulness meditation encourages the practitioner to observe wandering thoughts as they drift through the mind. The intention is not to get involved with the thoughts or to judge them, but simply to be aware of each mental note as it arises.

Through mindfulness meditation, you can see how your thoughts and feelings tend to move in particular patterns. Over time, you can become more aware of the human tendency to quickly judge an experience as good or bad, pleasant or unpleasant. With practice, an inner balance develops. What is mindfulness?

Mindfulness is the basic human ability to be fully present, aware of where we are and what we're doing, and not overly reactive or overwhelmed by what's going on around us.

While mindfulness is something, we all naturally possess, it's more readily available to us when we practice daily.

Whenever you bring awareness to what you're directly experiencing via your senses, or to your state of mind via your thoughts and emotions, you're being mindful. And there's growing research showing that when you train your brain to be mindful, you're remodelling the physical structure of your brain.

The goal of mindfulness is to wake up to the inner workings of our mental, emotional, and physical processes.

How do I practice mindfulness and meditation?

Mindfulness is available to us in every moment, whether through meditations and body scans, or mindful moment practises like taking time to pause and breathe when the phone rings instead of rushing to answer it.

Vipassana

Satyanarayan Goenka teaches a meditation technique given by the Buddha. It involves observing the sensations on the body. He calls it Vipassana. They have 10-day courses at their centres all over the world where this meditation is taught free of cost, step-by-step each day. These centres run on the generous donations given as gratitude by ex-students who have benefited hugely from these courses. You can enrol yourself at www.dhamma.org

I'm not writing down the steps here because it is best to learn from a teacher trained by S.N. Goenka.

Progressive Muscle Relaxation (PMR)

Steps to Practice Progressive Muscle Relaxation

Find a quiet place free from distractions. Lie on the floor or recline in a chair, loosen any tight clothing, and remove glasses or contacts. Rest your hands in your lap or on the arms of the chair. Take a few slow even breaths.

Now, focus your attention on the following areas, being careful to leave the rest of your body relaxed.

Forehead. Squeeze the muscles in your forehead, holding for 15 seconds. Feel the muscles becoming tighter and tenser. Then, slowly release the tension in your forehead while counting for 30 seconds. Notice the difference in how your muscles feel and the sensation of relaxation. Continue to release the tension until your forehead feels completely relaxed. Continue breathing slowly and evenly.

Jaw. Tense the muscles in your jaw, holding for 15 seconds. Then release the tension slowly while counting for 30 seconds. Notice the feeling of relaxation and continue to breathe slowly and evenly.

Neck and shoulders. Increase tension in your neck and shoulders by raising your shoulders toward your ears and hold for 15 seconds. Slowly release the tension as you count for 30 seconds. Notice the tension melting away.

Arms and hands. Slowly draw both hands into fists. Pull your fists into your chest and hold for 15 seconds, squeezing as tight as you can. Then slowly release while you count for 30 seconds. Notice the feeling of relaxation.

Buttocks. Slowly increase tension in your buttocks over 15 seconds. Then, slowly release the tension over 30 seconds. Notice the tension melting away. Continue to breathe slowly and evenly.

Legs. Slowly increase the tension in your quadriceps and calves over 15 seconds. Squeeze the muscles as hard as you can. Then gently release the tension over 30 seconds. Notice the tension melting away and the feeling of relaxation that is left.

Feet. Slowly increase the tension in your feet and toes. Tighten the muscles as much as you can. Then slowly release the tension while you count for 30 seconds. Notice all the tension melting away. Continue breathing slowly and evenly.

Enjoy the feeling of relaxation sweeping through your body. Continue to breathe slowly and evenly. This technique works well when you feel stressed and want to relax

Lake, Mountain, and Tree Meditations by Jon Kabat Zinn

Visualisations play a vital role in enriching and deepening your meditative experience. A good thing about visualisation is that one can be in any posture or be doing one's daily activities and yet enter into a meditative experience.

Jon Kabat-Zinn has introduced many such visualisation tools that we can make instrumental in enhancing our meditative experience.

Mountain Meditation

Mountains are elementally rock solid that represent a resolute determination to a practitioner of meditation. Like mountains sore the skies and yet are deeply rooted into the ground that they stand upon, so too, a practitioner can progress in her practice and yet be rooted in the fragile but tenacious reality of one's life. But this fragility is exactly what, with a strong determination like a firm and stable mountain, a practitioner is determined to transcend. Jon Kabat-Zinn in his beautiful technique teaches us how to borrow the qualities of a mountain in resolving to ourselves in bringing an inner change with a quintessentially emblematic quality of a mountain of abiding presence and stillness.

Instructions

This meditation is normally done in a sitting position, either on the floor or a chair, and begins by sensing into the support you have from the chair or the cushion, paying attention to the actual sensations of contact.

Finding a position of stability and poise, upper body balanced over your hips and shoulders in a comfortable but alert posture, hands on your lap or your knees, arms hanging by their own weight, like heavy curtains, stable and relaxed.

Actually, sensing into your body, feeling your feet… legs… hips… lower and upper body… arms… shoulders… neck… head…

And when you are ready, allowing your eyes to close, bringing awareness to the breath, the actual physical sensations, feeling each breath as it comes in and goes out… letting the breath be just as it is, without trying to change or regulate it in any way… allowing it to flow easily and naturally, with its own rhythm and pace, knowing you are breathing perfectly well right now, nothing for you to do…

Allowing the body to be still and sitting with a sense of dignity, a sense of resolve, a sense of being complete, whole, in this very moment, with your posture reflecting this sense of wholeness… (long pause)

As you sit here, letting an image form in your mind's eye, of the most magnificent or beautiful mountain you know or have seen or can imagine…, letting it gradually come into greater focus… and even if it doesn't come as a visual image, allowing the sense of this mountain and feeling its overall shape, its lofty peak or peaks high in the sky, the large base rooted in the bedrock of the earth's crust, it's steep or gently sloping sides...

Noticing how massive it is, how solid, how unmoving, how beautiful, whether from afar or up close...(pause)

Perhaps your mountain has snow blanketing its top and trees reaching down to the base, or rugged granite sides... there may be streams and waterfalls cascading down the slopes... there may be one peak or a series of peaks, or with meadows and high lakes...

Observing it, noting its qualities and when you feel ready, seeing if you can bring the mountain into your own body sitting here so that your body and the mountain in your mind's eye become one so that as you sit here, you share in the massiveness and the stillness and majesty of the mountain, you become the mountain.

Grounded in the sitting posture, your head becomes the lofty peak, supported by the rest of the body and affording a panoramic view. Your shoulders and arms the sides of the mountain. Your buttocks and legs the solid base, rooted to your cushion or your chair, experiencing in your body a sense of uplift from deep within your pelvis and spine.

With each breath, as you continue sitting, becoming a little more a breathing mountain, alive and vital, yet unwavering in your inner stillness, completely what you are, beyond words and thoughts, a centred, grounded, unmoving presence...

As you sit here, becoming aware of the fact that as the sun travels across the sky, the light and shadows and colours are changing virtually moment by moment in the mountain's stillness, and the surface teems with life and activity... streams, melting snow, waterfalls, plants and wildlife.

As the mountain sits, seeing and feeling how night follows day and day follows night. The bright warming sun, followed by the cool night sky studded with stars, and the gradual dawning of a new day...

Through it all, the mountain just sits, experiencing the change in each moment, constantly changing, yet always just being itself. It remains still as the seasons flow into one another and as the weather changes moment by moment and day by day, calmness abiding all change...

In summer, there is no snow on the mountain except perhaps for the very peaks or in crags shielded from direct sunlight

In the fall, the mountain may wear a coat of brilliant fire colours.

In winter, a blanket of snow and ice.

In any season, it may find itself at times enshrouded in clouds or fog or pelted by freezing rain. People may come to see the mountain and comment on how beautiful it is or how it's not a good day to see the mountain, that it's too cloudy or rainy or foggy or dark.

None of these matter to the mountain, which remains at all times its essential self. Clouds may come and clouds may go, tourists may like it or not. The mountain's magnificence and beauty are not changed one bit by whether people see it or not, seen or unseen, in sun or clouds, broiling or frigid, day or night.

It just sits, being itself.

At times visited by violent storms, buffeted by snow and rain and winds of unthinkable magnitude.

Through it all, the mountain sits.

Spring comes, trees leaf out, flowers bloom in the high meadows and slopes, birds sing in the trees once again. Streams overflow with the waters of melting snow.

Through it all, the mountain continues to sit, unmoved by the weather, by what happens on its surface, by the world of appearances... remaining its essential self, through the seasons, the changing weather, the activity ebbing and flowing on its surface...

In the same way, as we sit in meditation, we can learn to experience the mountain, we can embody the same central, unwavering stillness and groundedness in the face of everything that changes in our own lives, over seconds, over hours, over years.

In our lives and our meditation practice, we experience constantly the changing nature of mind and body and the outer world, we have our periods of light and darkness, activity and inactivity, our moments of colour and our moments of drabness.

We indeed experience storms of varying intensity and violence in the outer world and our minds and bodies, buffeted by high winds, by cold and rain, we endure periods of darkness and pain, as well as the moments of joy and uplift, even our appearance changes constantly, experiencing weather of its own...

By becoming the mountain in our meditation practice, we can link up with its strength and stability and adopt them for our own. We can use its energies to support our energy to encounter each moment with mindfulness and equanimity and clarity.

It may help us to see that our thoughts and feelings, our preoccupations, our emotional storms and crises, even the things that happen to us are very much like the weather on the mountain. We tend to take it all personally, but its strongest characteristic is impersonal.

The weather of our own lives is not be ignored or denied, it is to be encountered, honoured, felt, known for what it is, and held in awareness... And in holding it in this way, we come to know a deeper silence and stillness and wisdom.

Mountains have this to teach us and much more if we can let it in...

So if you find you resonate in some way with the strength and stability of the mountain in your sitting, it may be helpful to use it from time to time in your meditation practice, to remind you of what it means to sit mindfully with resolve and with wakefulness, in true stillness...

Continuing to sustain the mountain meditation on your own, in silence, moment by moment, for as long as you are comfortable.

Lake Meditation

Lake as a body of flowing water has a serenity to it. It also has a lot of vibrance which is undisturbed by any obstacle that comes its way. Water is as elemental as a rock but is stronger because it wears down the rock.

When we talk about overcoming obstacles, we are primarily talking about the thoughts that our mind is crowded with, while we meditate. Our mind should be like Water exhibiting the quality of taking in this 'information' and yet be in a continuous resuming mode showing our determination of overcoming this obstacle and staying our ground. A strong determination, a continuous flow in ourselves, is what will give us results in our meditational endeavour.

Script

This meditation is done mainly in a lying or reclining position, and begins by paying attention to the actual sensations of contact and support as you lie down, noticing where your body is making contact, how your weight is distributed on the floor, bed or recliner… sensing into your body, feeling your feet… your legs… hips… lower and upper body… arms… your shoulders and your head…

And when you are ready, bringing awareness to the breath, the actual physical sensations, feeling each breath as it comes in and goes out… letting the breath be just as it is, without trying to change or regulate it in any way… allowing it to flow easily and naturally, with its own rhythm and pace, knowing you are breathing perfectly well right now, nothing for you to do, allowing a sense of being complete, whole, in this very moment, just letting your breath be your breath…

As you rest here, letting an image form in your mind's eye of a lake, a body of water, large or small, held in a receptive basin by the earth itself, noting in the mind's eye and your own heart, that water likes to pool in low places, it seeks its own level, asks to be held, contained.

Letting this image gradually come into greater focus. Even if it doesn't come as a visual image, allowing the sense of this lake and feeling its presence…

The lake you're invoking may be deep or shallow, blue or green, muddy or clear. With no wind, the surface will be flat, mirror-like, reflecting trees rocks, sky and clouds, holding everything in itself momentarily...

Wind may come and stir up waves, causing the reflections to distort and disappear, but then sunlight may sparkle in the ripples and dance on the waves in a play of shimmering diamonds...

When night comes, it's the moon's turn to dance on the lake, or when the surface is still, to be reflected in it along with the outline of trees and shadows. In winter, the lake may freeze over, yet be teeming with movement and life below...

As you rest here breathing, as you establish this image of a lake in your mind's eye, allowing yourself, when you feel ready, to bring it inside yourself completely, so that your being merges with the lake, becomes one with it, so that all your energies in this moment are held in awareness with openness and compassion for yourself, in the same way as the lake's waters are held by the receptive and accepting basin of the earth herself.

Breathing as the lake, feeling its body as your body, allowing your mind and your heart to be open and receptive, moment by moment, to reflect whatever comes near, or to be clear all the way to the bottom. Experiencing moments of complete stillness, when both reflection and water are completely clear...and other moments perhaps when the surface is disturbed, choppy, stirred up, reflections and depth lost for the moment.

And through it all, as you lie here, simply observing the play of the various energies of your mind and heart, the fleeting thoughts and feelings, impulses and reactions, which come and go as ripples and waves, noting their effects. In contact with them, just as you are in contact with and feel the various changing energies that play on the lake, the wind, the waves, the light, the shadows and the reflections, the colours and smells.

Noticing the effect of your thoughts and feelings. Do they disturb the surface and clarity of the mind's lake? Do they muddy the waters? Is that okay with you? Isn't having a rippling or a wavy surface a part of being a lake? Might it be possible to identify not only with the surface of your lake but with the entire body of water, so that you become the stillness below the surface as well, which at most experiences only gentle undulations, even when the surface is choppy and ragged?

And in the same way, in your meditation practice and your daily life, can you be in touch, not only with the changing content and intensity of your thoughts and feelings but also with the vast unwavering reservoir of awareness itself, residing below the surface of your mind. The lake can teach this, remind us of the lake within ourselves.

If you find this image to be of value, you may want to use it from time to time to deepen and enrich your meditation practice. You might also invite this lake image to empower you and guide your actions in the world as you move through the unfolding of each day, carrying this vast reservoir of mindfulness within your heart...

Dwelling here in the stillness of this moment, until signalled by the sound of the bells, we can be the lake in silence now, affirming our ability to hold in awareness and acceptance, right now, all our qualities of mind and body, just as the lake sits held, cradled, contained by the earth, reflecting sun, moon, stars, trees, clouds and sky, birds and light, caressed by the air and the wind, which bring out and highlight its sparkle, its vitality, its potential, moment by moment.

Continue to sustain the lake meditation on your own for as long as you are comfortable, in silence, moment by moment, being the lake with its storms and moments of peace.

Tree Meditation

Standing meditation is best learned from trees. If possible, stand close to one or under it. If not stand anywhere you find convenient. Feel your feet developing roots into the ground. Feel your body sway gently, as it always will, just as trees do in a breeze. Staying put, in touch with your breathing, drink in what is in front of you, or keep your eyes closed and sense your surroundings. Sense the tree closest to you. Listen to it, feel its presence, touch it with your mind and body.

Use your breath to help you to stay in the moment...feeling your own body standing, breathing, being, moment by moment.

When mind or body first signals that perhaps it is time to move on, stay with the standing a while longer, remembering that trees stand still for years, occasionally lifetimes if they are fortunate. See if they do not have something to teach you about stillness and about being in touch. After all, they are touching the ground with roots and trunk, the air with trunk and branches, sunlight and the wind with their leaves; everything about a standing tree speaks of being in touch. Experiment with standing this way yourself, even for short periods. Work at being in touch with the air on your skin, the feel of the feet in contact with the ground, the sounds of the world, the dance of light and colour and shadow, the dance of the mind.

Standing like this wherever you find yourself, in the woods, in the mountains, by a river, in your living room, or just waiting for the bus. When you are alone, you might try opening your palms to the sky and holding your arms out in various positions, like branches and leaves, accessible, open, receptive, patient.

Thich Nhat Hanh's Walking Meditation

One of the strongest supporters of walking meditation, Thich Nhat Hanh says that every path, every street in the world is your walking meditation path. Walking meditation is practising meditation while walking. It can bring you joy and peace while you practice it.

Take short steps in complete relaxation; go slowly with a smile on your lips, with your heart open to an experience of peace. You can feel truly at ease with yourself. Your steps can be those of the healthiest, most secure person on earth. All sorrows and worries can drop away while you are walking. To have peace of mind, to attain self-liberation, learn to walk in this way. It is not difficult. You can do it. Anyone can do it who has some degree of mindfulness and a true intention to be happy.

There are varied forms of Walking Meditation out there like, Theravada Walking Meditation, Zen Walking Meditation, Mindfulness Walking Meditation, Yoga Walking Meditation, and Daoist Walking Meditation but, Thich Nhat Hanh's technique stands out for its simplicity in application.

Script

Walk slowly, with calmness and comfort

Be aware of each move, of each step. Keep bringing your attention to the present moment.

Mentally repeat one of these verses, as you walk

Breathing in "I have arrived"; Breathing out "I am home"

Breathing in "In the here"; Breathing out "In the now"

Breathing in "I am solid"; Breathing out "I am free"

Breathing in "In the ultimate"; Breathing out "I dwell"

Enjoy every step you take. Kiss the earth with your feet, imprinting gratitude and love as you walk.

Creative Visualization

What Is Creative Visualization?

Creative visualization is using the power of our mind to imagine the desired outcome. This meditation can be used to promote success in every area of our lives. Visualization is the process of putting together visual mental imagery of what you are wanting to manifest. Consequently, you can start to gain emotions associated with the desired image. In simpler terms, creative visualization is where you visualize what you want and experience the emotions or feelings you would have if it were true.

This can then help you to put your goals and desires out into the universe and start to feel motivated to achieve them. Much like a vision board, but the imagery is in your mind, not physical, although both creative visualization and a physical vision board have very similar purposes.

Creative Visualization can be extremely powerful as you are using the mind's eye to create detailed images of what you want to manifest. This can help you to feel more positive and motivated to achieve these goals. After visualizing, you should feel inspired and ready to take action towards your goals.

If you are constantly repeating certain thoughts to yourself, your subconscious mind accepts these thoughts and this causes a change in your long-term mindset.

This change in mindset can then have a knock-on effect on your behaviours, feelings, and habits. And this is the reason why creative visualization can be so effective!

The mind is a very powerful thing and the visual images that are created through creative visualization can determine some of the strong feelings and emotions that you experience when you think of them. This is why it's important to be clear about what you want to visualize and why.

You can use creative visualization to help you achieve and manifest the outcomes that you desire. These thoughts can be repeated in your mind, which should help to change your mindset and ultimately, your behaviour, in a way that is geared towards your goals.

Lastly, creative visualization can also be used for a therapeutic application. This is where visual imagery can be used to replace and recreate images that are upsetting or cause stress.

Benefits of Creative Visualization Techniques

Now that you know the basics of what visualization is, let's take a deeper look at the benefits. Creative Visualization techniques can offer many benefits and it can do much more than just help you with your manifestations.

Here are 6 benefits of Creative Visualization techniques.

1. Busts Stress

Creative Visualization has shown that positive visual mental images help to increase physical and mental relaxation and decrease stress. Even just taking the time out of your day to be still, silent and relaxed when visualizing can help to reduce your stress and help you feel more positive. Visualization is a form of relaxation just like any other meditation.

Because you would normally be visualizing positive situations, it can naturally help to quieten your mind and keep you feeling relaxed.

2. Develops Focus

You can increase your focus and concentration by sitting down and visualizing. When you perform a task such as creative visualization you are forgetting your troubles from the day and any worries you might have about the future. This gives you a chance to just focus and concentrate on your visualizations.

3. Gain Self Confidence

When you visualize, you are normally picturing yourself achieving success and experiencing positive situations. This means that your self-confidence can increase, as you would be starting to believe in yourself and that your visualizations could come true. The more you visualize yourself doing amazing things, the more confident in yourself you can become.

4. Brings You Joy

Even though the visualization may not be true right now, even the thought of it can spark joy in your life. This is because your mind won't know the difference between the visualization and doing that thing.

This means that you can experience the joy and excitement you would feel if it were real, which only makes your visualizations stronger.

5. Gives You Inspiration

Just like with our confidence, visualizations can also give us a big dose of inspiration. When we visualize our goals and dreams, we become inspired to make them happen. This inspiration can spur us to take action toward our goals.

If we can see our goals in a visualization then it inspires us to make sure we will see it in our reality as well.

6. Improved Relationships

As creative visualization can help you with positivity, motivation, confidence, and inspiration, it can also help you with improved relationships. This could be with friends or a partner.

As you visualize you become more confident in yourself and your abilities. This can help to improve your social life and relationships as your overall wellbeing will be improved.

Six Steps to Begin Using Creative Visualization

Are you looking for your dream job? Or maybe you are on the search for a suitable partner or wondering how you can develop more self-confidence... Now you know the reasons to start using visualization in your manifestation practice, we can take a deeper delve into how to use creative visualization in practice.

Whatever your goal, be sure to try these basic steps to start using creative visualization to your advantage.

Step One: Set the Mood

It is vital to be in a relaxed and positive state of mind when you attempt creative visualization. For example, you might try taking a quiet walk in a peaceful area, soaking in a hot bath or listening to mellow instrumental music.

Once you're feeling relaxed, find a place where you won't be disturbed and can be comfortable for the duration of the process. The longer you can spend working on your visualization, the more effective it is likely to be.

Step Two: Enter A Meditative State

Creative visualization tends to be most intense and meaningful if you take the time to do a straightforward meditative exercise before you begin. For most people, all that is needed is a few minutes spent focusing on slow, steady breathing.

Step Three: Visualize Your Goal

Once your mind feels still and receptive, start crafting an image of the thing you want, taking as long as you like to build up all of the details.

For example, if you are working towards a major promotion at work, imagine yourself receiving the announcement and picture the positive reactions of people around you.

Try to make the environment as realistic as possible, and do your best to experience not just the sights but also the sounds, scents and tactile sensations associated with your goal.

Step Four: Hold onto The Feelings Associated with Your Visualization

Although the most important part of creative visualization is the process described in step three, you are more likely to see your goals manifest in your life if you allow your visualization experiences to influence the rest of your day.

Try to hold onto the feelings of pride, happiness, confidence, and peace that you experience when you picture your goal, and repeatedly affirm your belief that you will soon attract the things you yearn for.

Step Five: Make A Habit of Using Creative Visualization

Ideally, you should make creative visualization a daily part of your life. Most people find it useful to set aside a specific time for the visualization (such as fifteen minutes before going to sleep), but the most important thing is that you maintain your ritual of visualizing your goal until you obtain what you want in your life.

Step Six: Work Hard to Achieve Your Goal

Although creative visualization is incredibly powerful and can certainly play a huge role in allowing you to develop the life you've always wanted, you substantially increase your chances of success if you also take concrete steps towards your goals.

Take every relevant opportunity you encounter, be brave, and believe in a happier, more fulfilling life.

You can try all of these methods, and choose one which suits you best. Once you have made a choice practise it daily for at least for ninety days to see significant results.

Chapter Six

Take Charge

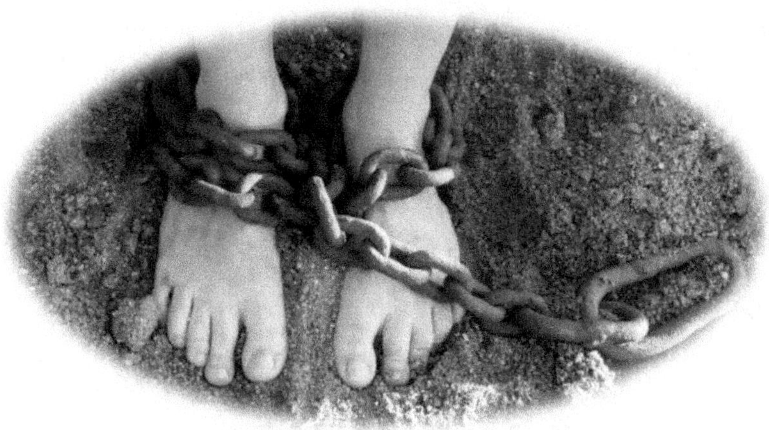

All said and done the million-dollar question to be asked to oneself remains, which is, "Do I really want to be happy?" You might think this to be an absurd question. You might say "Why would I even read a self-help book on happiness if I did not want to be happy."

Wait! Before you get annoyed at me, take a moment close your eyes, and be still. Think to yourself "Do I have some advantages in being miserable?". Think about all aspects of your life. Family, friends, social, religious, career, etc.

Charles Dickens wrote about a prisoner who was locked up for many years in a dungeon. After serving his sentence, he got his freedom. He was brought out from his cell into the bright daylight of the open world. This man looked all around and after a few moments, was so uncomfortable with his newly acquired freedom, that he asked to be taken back to the confines of his cell. To him, the jail, the fetters, and the darkness were more familiar, secure, and, comfortable than accepting the change of freedom and an open world.

Human nature generally resists change. Change is uncomfortable. Regardless of its positive or negative effect, change can often be stressful. Sometimes we get so comfortable with our negativity that even when the change is for the better, we don't want to accept it.

I love this story from the Bible. A man lay helplessly by the pool of Bethesda. This wasn't just any pool. It was rumoured that angels came periodically and stirred the water, and whoever dived in first received miraculous healing. Needless to say, people flocked from near and far for a chance to participate in the phenomenon.

However, this one man, sick for thirty-eight years, could never make it to the pool fast enough. It was a bit of a hopeless situation for him.

One day Jesus sees him lying there and knows that he has already been there for a long time. He says to him, "Do you want to be healed?"

You might think this to be a ridiculous question because obviously, he wants to be healed.

Or, does he really?

It's fascinating that when the sick man answered Jesus, he didn't give a simple yes or no. He offered an excuse. "Sir, I have no one to put me into the pool when the water is stirred up, and while I am going someone steps down before me."

Think about it. This man has been sick for thirty-eight years. He's comfortable in his disease by this point. He's resigned himself to being the victim and blaming others. He's having a pity-pool-party.

"Do you want to be healed?". "Do you want to be happy"

Resignation is a dangerous thing.

Jesus gave this man back a sense of purpose. He freed him from the bonds of self-pity, pride, fear, discouragement, hopelessness, and resignation, all in one amazingly-effective command.

"Get up, take up your bed, and walk."

What? How? He hadn't even gone into the water yet.

Jesus had invited the man into his own healing process.

Now think about your misery as a sickness. Your emotional wound. Your scar. Your grudge. Your bitterness. Your unforgiveness. That disease that you've formed around you like a wall, effectively keeping out any additional pain and suffering.

You've got used to it. It's like a security blanket. It's scratchy, dirty and damp, but it's your protection now. You talk about getting rid of this blanket, how it's awful, and stinks, and you're so desperate to be free of it. But when anyone tries to tug it away, you hold on tight.

Do you really want to be happy?

Notice how the sick man had resigned himself to lingering near the healing, but not participating in it. How often do we do that? We read self- help books, take coaching, counselling, and therapy. We learn everything there is to learn about happiness. We know the drawbacks of staying unhappy and the benefits of becoming happy.

Maybe that's why Jesus asked him "Do you want to be healed?" He already knew the answer.

But the sick man needed to know the answer.

He needed to participate in his own healing. He needed to face the fact that sometimes, healing can be dangerous. It can even hurt worse than the original wound. Broken bones have to be set. And that setting can first mean re-breaking.

But it's the difference between living your life pool-side, and swimming freely in the abundant sea of happiness. This is the choice you will need to make.

This is not a prescriptive or a directive book. I am not a psychologist. This book is based on my own meandering experiences and tried and tested methods gathered from fellow seekers or masters. What worked for me may not work for you. I do not take credit for any of the methods suggested here. I am just a compiler of methods that I have experienced, practised, and suggested.

Read the book and try out for yourself the remedies given. Discard the ones which do not resonate with you. Continue practising the ones which work for you. In time you might find something else which makes you happy. Or you might find a completely new way of becoming happy. Do it. Don't sit by the poolside. Take a plunge into the rejuvenating lake. Take ownership of your own mental wellbeing.

Let's do this powerful exercise:

Think of all the good things being in an unhappy state will bring to you. You might say "How can there be anything good about being in an unhappy state?" Think deeply. These things are on a subconscious level and we are not even aware of the fact that we have chosen to be unhappy as a coping mechanism. Or to fulfil some underlying emotional need and thus we attract experiences which make us unhappy.

Once you understand this, you can find some other positive ways to satisfy this need and won't need the crutches of unhappiness. You could have unconsciously chosen an unhappy state of mind as a self-imposed punishment for some guilt you are carrying or somewhere, sometime the belief that you are cared for by your loved ones only when you are sad, is reinforced in your mind. Or you might have become addicted to the sympathy shown by people to you when you are unhappy. It also could be that you are afraid that people will not like you if you become unhappy.

Once upon a time, I suffered from all of these beliefs and I was not at all aware of it. Once you are aware of the root cause of your unhappiness, it is easy to treat it. It is like a diagnosis. Once you know the disease, treatment goes in the right direction. Self-awareness is the first step towards healing. Look at the picture of, 'The wheel of life' given below. List down how you staying in an unhappy state all the time, will impact each component of this wheel

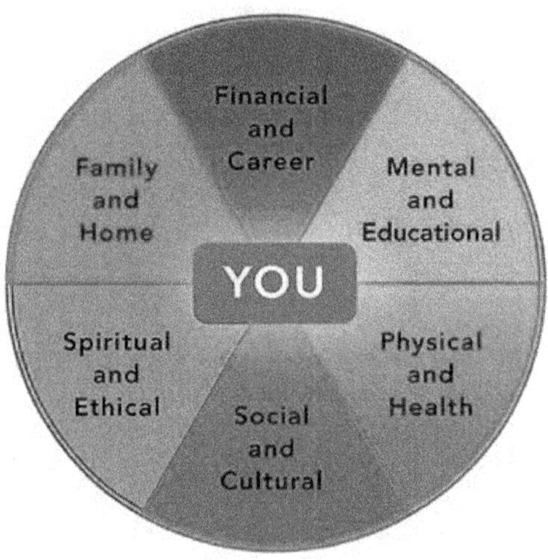

Now make a list of all the good things that happiness can bring into your life. Look at the picture of 'The wheel of life again. List down how happiness will impact every component of this wheel. Make this list as detailed as possible Write down at least ten things that will change in each component of the wheel.

Now think of your life five years from now, if you remain unhappy. Take a sheet of paper and draw a picture of your life the way it would look, if you continue being miserable. Make the picture detailed. Add all the pains and the perceived benefits. Draw and paint all the aspects of your miserable life five years from now if you continue to wallow in your misery.

Now think of your life five years from now if you become happy. Take a sheet of paper and draw a picture of your life the way it would look, if you strive to be happy consistently and mindfully. Make the picture detailed, colourful, and bright. Sketch all the people who you think will be with you. Draw all the places you think you will go to. If you don't like to draw you can make a collage by cutting off pictures from magazines or download from the internet. Make this into a large poster, detailed and colourful and bright.

Now look at both the pictures and choose the one you really wish your future to look like. Definitely it will be the second one. The beautiful joyous one! Take action from today to realise the picture. Be brave enough to break the

Fit as a Fiddle Happy as a Lark

mind binders, the self-made fetters those bind you to misery.

Imagination without action is like daydreaming and waiting for things to happen automatically.

So, take charge and move forward to discover your true and happy self!

**"What we are today comes
from our thoughts of yesterday,
and present thoughts build
our life of tomorrow:
our life is the creation of our own mind"**
— The Buddha